2023

Selected 2022 Articles from
The Medical Letter on Drugs and Therapeutics®

Published by

The Medical Letter, Inc.
145 Huguenot St., Ste. 312
New Rochelle, New York 10801-7537

800-211-2769
914-235-0500
Fax 914-632-1733
www.medicalletter.org

24th Edition

The Medical Letter, Inc.
145 Huguenot St., Ste. 312
New Rochelle, New York 10801-7537

Contents

Tables

Weight Management

Introduction

The Medical Letter, Inc. is a nonprofit organization that publishes critical appraisals of new prescription drugs and comparative reviews of drugs for common diseases in its newsletter, *The Medical Letter on Drugs and Therapeutics*. It is committed to providing objective, practical, and timely information on drugs and treatments of common diseases to help readers make the best decisions for their patients—without the influence of the pharmaceutical industry. The Medical Letter is supported by its readers, and does not receive any commercial support or accept advertising in any of its publications.

Many of our readers know that pharmaceutical companies and their representatives often exaggerate the therapeutic effects and understate the adverse effects of their products, but busy practitioners have neither the time nor the resources to check the accuracy of the manufacturers' claims. Our publication is intended specifically to meet the needs of busy healthcare professionals who want unbiased, reliable, and timely drug information. Our editorial process is designed to ensure that the information we provide represents an unbiased consensus of medical experts.

The editorial process used for *The Medical Letter on Drugs and Therapeutics* relies on a consensus of experts to develop prescribing recommendations. The first draft of an article is prepared by one of our in-house or contributing editors or by an outside expert. This initial draft is edited and sent to our Contributing Editors, to 10-20 other reviewers who have clinical and/or experimental experience with the drug or type of drug or disease under review, to the FDA, and to the first and last authors of all the articles cited in the text. Many critical observations, suggestions, and questions are received from the reviewers and are incorporated into the article during the revision process. Further communication as needed is followed by fact checking and editing to make sure the final appraisal is not only accurate, but also easy to read.

NOTE: The drug costs listed in the tables are based on the pricing information that was available in the month the article was originally published. When the cost of a drug has been updated or added since publication, it is designated as such.

The Medical Letter, Inc. is based in New Rochelle, NY. For more information, go to www.medicalletter.org or call 800-211-2769.

DRUGS FOR
Acute Otitis Media in Children

Original publication date – February 2022

More antibiotics are prescribed for treatment of acute otitis media (AOM) than for any other infection in young children. Children with AOM typically present with otalgia, fever, and bulging and erythema of the tympanic membrane.

CAUSATIVE PATHOGENS — Before universal infant vaccination with pneumococcal conjugate vaccines began in the early 2000s, *Streptococcus pneumoniae* was the most common bacterial pathogen associated with AOM in children; it now accounts for ≤25% of cases, and the serotypes that now cause AOM in children often have reduced susceptibility to amoxicillin. *Haemophilus influenzae* is now the most frequently isolated bacterial pathogen. In a recent study, about half of the *H. influenzae* strains isolated from children with AOM produced beta-lactamase and were resistant to amoxicillin.[1] *Moraxella catarrhalis*, which also produces beta-lactamase and is resistant to amoxicillin, is the third-most frequently isolated bacterial pathogen in children with AOM.[1,2] Group A streptococcus, *Staphylococcus aureus*, and anaerobic bacteria are less common causes. AOM is also frequently associated with viral respiratory infections.

STANDARD TREATMENT — Oral ibuprofen or acetaminophen should be used to reduce otalgia in children with AOM.

Drugs for Acute Otitis Media in Children

> **Key Points: Treatment of Acute Otitis Media in Children**
>
> ▶ Nontypeable *Haemophilus influenzae* is now the most common causative pathogen of acute otitis media (AOM) in children.
>
> ▶ All children <2 years old and older children with severe infection (i.e., otorrhea, otalgia for more than 48 hours, or a temperature ≥102.2°F) should receive immediate antibiotic treatment for AOM.
>
> ▶ High-dose amoxicillin has been used for treatment of AOM in children for years, but because of the increased prevalence of AOM caused by beta-lactamase producing strains of *H. influenzae* and *M. catarrhalis*, some expert clinicians now recommend amoxicillin-clavulanate for initial treatment.
>
> ▶ Amoxicillin-clavulanate is recommended for children who were recently treated with a beta-lactam antibiotic, those with a history of recurrent AOM unresponsive to amoxicillin, and those with concomitant purulent conjunctivitis.
>
> ▶ In all children with AOM, otalgia should be treated with oral acetaminophen or ibuprofen.

Antimicrobial therapy can shorten the duration of symptoms of AOM and prevent complications, but even without effective antibiotic treatment, severe symptoms generally last only a few days and most infections resolve on their own. Immediate antibiotic treatment should be prescribed for all children <2 years old, and for older children with severe infection (i.e., otorrhea, severe or persistent otalgia for more than 48 hours, or a temperature ≥102.2°F). In other cases, watchful waiting combined with analgesia is an appropriate treatment strategy; if symptoms fail to improve or worsen within 48-72 hours, antibiotic therapy should be started.

Most cases of AOM are treated empirically. Guidelines for treatment of AOM in children, which were last published in 2013, recommended high-dose amoxicillin (90 mg/kg/day) for initial treatment in most children. (The higher dose of amoxicillin is used to improve activity against strains of *S. pneumoniae* with reduced susceptibility to amoxicillin.) Amoxicillin-clavulanate (*Augmentin*, and generics) was recommended for initial treatment of children who were more likely to be infected with a beta-lactamase-producing strain of *H. influenzae* (i.e., those who were recently treated with a beta-lactam antibiotic, those with a history of recurrent AOM that was unresponsive to amoxicillin, and those with purulent conjunctivitis).[3]

High-dose amoxicillin is still considered by many to be the treatment of choice for most cases of AOM in children, but since the likelihood of infection with *S. pneumoniae* has declined with routine childhood immunization and the prevalence of beta-lactamase-producing *H. influenzae* has increased, some expert clinicians now recommend standard-dose amoxicillin-clavulanate (45 mg/kg/day of the amoxicillin component) for first-line treatment in all children without an allergy to penicillin.[2] Others prefer a high-dose of amoxicillin-clavulanate to also provide adequate coverage of strains of *S. pneumoniae* that have reduced susceptibility to amoxicillin.[4]

A cephalosporin (oral cefdinir, cefpodoxime, or cefuroxime, or IM/IV ceftriaxone) is recommended for patients with a history of penicillin allergy; the risk of cross-reactivity between penicillin or amoxicillin and later-generation cephalosporins is low.[5]

Macrolide antibiotics such as azithromycin (*Zithromax*, and generics) have limited activity against *S. pneumoniae* and *H. influenzae*; they should be considered only for patients with a history of serious penicillin allergy. Clindamycin may be effective for treatment of AOM caused by *S. pneumoniae*, but it has no activity against *H. influenzae* or *M. catarrhalis*.

TREATMENT FAILURE — Signs and symptoms of AOM should begin to resolve within 48-72 hours after initiation of antibiotic treatment, but middle ear effusion can persist for months after successful treatment. When symptoms and middle ear inflammation recur, another antibiotic should be selected. When a series of antibiotics has failed, tympanocentesis should be considered for bacteriologic susceptibility testing.

PREVENTION OF RECURRENCE — Antibiotic prophylaxis to reduce the frequency of infection in children is not recommended.

Table 1. Initial Treatment of Acute Otitis Media in Children		
Drug	**Dosage**	**Duration**[1]
Amoxicillin	90 mg/kg/day PO in 2 divided doses (max 4000 mg/day)	5-10 days
OR		
Amoxicillin- clavulanic acid[2]	90-6.4 mg/kg/day PO in 2 divided doses (max 4000 mg/day of amoxicillin)[3]	5-10 days
Alternatives (penicillin allergy)		
Cefdinir	14 mg/kg/day PO in 1 or 2 doses (max 600 mg/day)	5-10 days
Cefpodoxime	10 mg/kg/day PO in 2 divided doses (max 200 mg/dose)	5-10 days
Cefuroxime	30 mg/kg/day PO in 2 divided doses (max 500 mg/dose)	5-10 days
Ceftriaxone	50 mg/kg/day IM or IV (max 1000 mg/day)	1-3 days

1. In children <2 years old or with severe symptoms, a 10-day course is recommended. A 5- to-7-day course may be equally effective in older children with mild to moderate symptoms.
2. Because of the increased prevalence of AOM caused by beta-lactamase-producing organisms (*M. catarrhalis* and about half of *H. influenzae* strains), some expert clinicians now recommend amoxicillin-clavulanate for initial treatment in all patients. The addition of clavulanic acid restores amoxicillin's activity against organisms that produce beta-lactamase. Amoxicillin-clavulanate is preferred for children who have received amoxicillin in the past 30 days or have a history of recurrent AOM that was unresponsive to amoxicillin. Concomitant purulent conjunctivitis may indicate infection with *H. influenzae*; amoxicillin-clavulanate is also recommended for initial treatment in these patients.
3. 45 mg/kg/day of amoxicillin is an alternative; this dose is less likely to be effective for AOM caused by strains of *S. pneumoniae* with reduced susceptibility to amoxicillin.

Tympanostomy tubes can be considered for children with recurrent AOM (≥3 episodes of AOM within 6 months or 4 episodes within one year with one episode in the preceding 6 months). However, in one clinical trial in 250 children 6 to 35 months old with recurrent AOM, the rate of episodes during a 2-year period was not significantly lower in children who underwent tympanostomy tube placement than in those who were managed with episodic antibiotic treatment.[6]

ADVERSE EFFECTS — All antibacterial agents used to treat children for AOM can cause diarrhea, vomiting, and rash. Amoxicillin-clavulanate and cephalosporin antibiotics cause a higher incidence of diarrhea than amoxicillin.

1. R Kaur et al. Dynamic changes in otopathogens colonizing the nasopharynx and causing acute otitis media in children after 13-valent (PCV-13) pneumococcal conjugate vaccination during 2015-2019. Eur J Clin Microbiol Infect Dis 2022; 41:37.
2. ER Wald and GP DeMuri. Antibiotic recommendations for acute otitis media and acute bacterial sinusitis: conundrum no more. Pediatr Infect Dis J 2018; 37:1255.
3. AS Lieberthal et al. Clinical practice guideline: the diagnosis and management of acute otitis media. Pediatrics 2013; 131:e964.
4. ME Pichichero. Considering an otitis media antibiotic change. J Pediatr 2020; 222:253.
5. RJ Zagursky and ME Pichichero. Cross-reactivity in β-lactam allergy. J Allergy Clin Immunol Pract 2018; 6:72.
6. A Hoberman et al. Tympanostomy tubes or medical management for recurrent otitis media. N Engl J Med 2021; 384:1789.

| Adult Immunization

Original publication date – October 2022

The Advisory Committee on Immunization Practices (ACIP) recommends use of certain vaccines in adults residing in the US.[1] Routine childhood immunization has reduced the overall incidence of some of these vaccine-preventable diseases, but many adults remain susceptible. Recommendations for vaccination against COVID-19, seasonal influenza, and monkeypox and vaccination of travelers have been reviewed separately.[2-5]

TETANUS, DIPHTHERIA, AND PERTUSSIS — Administration of a tetanus, diphtheria, and pertussis vaccine has been part of routine childhood immunization since the 1940s. Vaccines containing tetanus and diphtheria toxoids (Td) without pertussis have been used for many years as a booster dose for adults, but pertussis infection can occur when vaccine-induced immunity has waned over time and infected parents and siblings have transmitted pertussis to unimmunized and under immunized infants. Vaccines containing tetanus and diphtheria toxoids combined with protein components of acellular pertussis (Tdap; *Adacel*, *Boostrix*) are now recommended for use in adults.

Recommendations – Adults with an uncertain history of primary vaccination should receive 3 doses of a Td-containing vaccine, one of which (preferably the first) should be Tdap. The first 2 doses should be administered at least 4 weeks apart and the third dose 6-12 months after the second. Any adult who has never received a dose of Tdap should receive one as soon as possible, regardless of the interval since the last Td-containing vaccine. A Td or Tdap booster should be given every 10 years.[6]

Pregnant women should receive Tdap during each pregnancy, regardless of the interval since the last Td or Tdap vaccination, to protect the newborn against pertussis in the first months of life. The vaccine should be given during the early part of gestational weeks 27 through 36 to maximize the transfer of maternal antibodies.[6] Pregnant women with an uncertain or incomplete history of primary vaccination should be given 3 doses of a Td-containing vaccine, one of which should be Tdap. Women who have never received Tdap and did not receive it during pregnancy should be vaccinated immediately postpartum.

Adverse Effects – Injection-site reactions are common with administration of Td or Tdap, but they are usually mild. Fever and injection-site pain have been more frequent with Tdap than with Td. Arthus-type reactions with extensive painful swelling have occurred rarely in adults with a history of repeated vaccinations.

MEASLES, MUMPS, AND RUBELLA (MMR) — Importation of measles by international travelers has led to outbreaks in the US, primarily in unvaccinated persons. During the COVID-19 pandemic, there has been a marked reduction in administration of measles-containing vaccine, resulting in a growing population that may be susceptible to measles.[7] Sporadic mumps outbreaks, mainly in fully vaccinated adolescents and young adults, also continue to occur on college campuses and in other congregate settings.[8]

The MMR vaccine contains live-attenuated viruses; measles and mumps viruses are both derived from chick embryo cell culture and rubella virus is derived from human diploid cell culture.

Recommendations – Adults born in the US before 1957 (1970 in Canada) can be considered immune to measles, mumps, and rubella. Most other adults who lack evidence of immunity (documentation of vaccination, laboratory evidence of immunity, previously vaccinated with the killed [or an unknown] measles vaccine used from 1963 to 1967) should receive one dose of MMR vaccine. Two doses of the vaccine, separated by at least 28 days, are recommended for adults without evidence of immunity who are at high risk of exposure to or transmission of measles or mumps, including students in postsecondary educational institutions, international travelers, and household contacts of immunocompromised persons.[9] Healthcare workers of any age should be evaluated for evidence of immunity. For control of a mumps outbreak in a setting with intense exposure, high attack rates, and evidence of ongoing transmission, one additional dose of MMR vaccine is recommended for those who previously received ≤2 doses.[10]

One dose of MMR vaccine should be administered to nonpregnant women of childbearing age who lack evidence of immunity to rubella. **Pregnant women** who do not have evidence of immunity to rubella should receive a dose of MMR vaccine postpartum, before discharge from the healthcare facility.

Adverse Effects – Pain and erythema at the injection site, fever, rash, and transient arthralgias (in about 25% of women) are common following MMR vaccination. Few adverse events have been reported after a third dose of MMR vaccine. Anaphylactic reactions and thrombocytopenic purpura occur rarely.[9]

Contraindications – Because MMR is a live vaccine, it is contraindicated in **pregnant women** and in adults with severe immunodeficiency. The vaccine should not be given to persons with a history of anaphylaxis caused by neomycin (*M-M-R II* and *Priorix*) or gelatin *(M-M-R II)*.

VARICELLA — Primary varicella infection can be more severe in adults than in children. The varicella vaccine contains live-attenuated varicella virus.

Adult Immunization

Table 1. Some Vaccines for Adults

Vaccines	Recommendations[1]
Tetanus, Diphtheria (Td)	
Tenivac (Sanofi)[3] *Tdvax* (Grifols)[3]	▸ Primary series for previously unvaccinated adults ▸ Booster dose of Td or Tdap every 10 years
Tetanus, Diphtheria, Acellular Pertussis (Tdap)	
Adacel (Sanofi)[3] *Boostrix* (GSK)[3]	▸ Single dose for adults who have never received a Tdap vaccine regardless of interval since last Td[4] ▸ Booster dose of Td or Tdap every 10 years
Measles, Mumps, Rubella (MMR)	
M-M-R II (Merck)[6] *Priorix* (GSK)[6]	▸ Adults born during or after 1957 (1970 in Canada) without evidence of immunity
Varicella (VAR)	
Varivax (Merck)[6]	▸ Adults born during or after 1980 without evidence of immunity
Zoster	
Shingrix (RZV; GSK)[3]	▸ Adults ≥50 years old including those with a previous episode of herpes zoster or previous use of the live-attenuated vaccine (*Zostavax*) ▸ Adults ≥19 years old who are or will be immunodeficient or immunosuppressed because of disease or therapy
Human Papillomavirus (HPV)	
Gardasil 9 (Merck)[3]	▸ Previously unvaccinated persons through age 26 years[9]

1. Based on ACIP-recommended age ranges, which may differ from FDA-approved age ranges for some vaccines. See text for detailed information on indications, contraindications, and risk factors.
2. Approximate private sector cost (including excise tax) for 1 dose as of July 1, 2022, according to the CDC Vaccine Price List. Available at: www.cdc.gov/vaccines/programs/vfc/awardees/vaccine-management/price-list/index.html?s_cid=cs_000. Accessed August 2022.
3. Inactivated vaccine.
4. Although *Adacel* is not FDA-licensed for persons ≥65 years old, the ACIP recommends use of either *Boostrix* or *Adacel* in persons ≥65 years old.
5. Pregnant women should receive Tdap during each pregnancy, ideally during the early part of gestational weeks 27-36.
6. Live-attenuated vaccine.
7. One to 2 doses for no evidence of immunity to measles and mumps (second dose must be administered at least 28 days after the first) and 1 dose for no evidence of immunity to rubella. One additional dose is recommended for adults who previously received ≤2 doses and are at risk for acquiring mumps because of an outbreak.

Usual Dose/Schedule	Cost[2]
0.5 mL IM/3 doses (0, 1, and 6-12 mos)	$37.90 27.20
0.5 mL IM/1 dose[5]	50.50 44.80
0.5 mL SC/1 or 2 doses[7]	87.30 85.10
0.5 mL SC/2 doses (0, 4-8 wks)	151.00
0.5 mL IM/2 doses (0, 2-6 mos)[8]	171.60
0.5 mL IM/3 doses (0, 1-2, and 6 mos)[10,11]	253.60

8. Immunocompromised patients who would benefit from a shorter schedule can be given the second dose 1-2 months after the first.
9. May be considered for some adults 27-45 years old who might be at risk of acquiring new HPV infections.
10. Minimum interval between doses 1 and 2 is 4 weeks, between doses 2 and 3 is 12 weeks, and between doses 1 and 3 is 5 months.
11. A 3-dose series is recommended for previously unvaccinated persons 15-26 years old. For those who started a series at age 9-14 years, but only received 1 dose or 2 doses <5 months apart, 1 additional dose is recommended.

Continued on next page

Table 1. Some Vaccines for Adults (continued)	
Vaccines	**Recommendations**[1]
Pneumococcal	
Prevnar 20 (PCV20; Pfizer)[3] *Vaxneuvance* (PCV15; Merck)[3] *Pneumovax 23* (PPSV23; Merck)[3]	▸ PCV20 **OR** PCV15 followed by PPSV23 ≥1 year later for previously unvaccinated adults ≥65 years old and for those <65 years old with specific risk factors (see Table 4)
Hepatitis A (HepA)	
Havrix (GSK)[3] *Vaqta* (Merck)[3]	▸ Previously unvaccinated adults with medical, occupational, or behavioral risk factors (see Table 5) or who lack a risk factor but want protection
Hepatitis B (HepB)	
Heplisav-B (Dynavax)[3] *Engerix-B* (GSK)[3] *Recombivax HB* (Merck)[3] *PreHevbrio* (VBI)[3]	▸ All persons ≤59 years old ▸ Previously unvaccinated adults ≥60 years old with medical, occupational, or behavioral risk factors (see Table 6) ▸ Should be offered to adults ≥60 years old who lack a risk factor
Hepatitis A/B (HepA/HepB)	
Twinrix (GSK)[3]	▸ Adults who require both HepA and HepB vaccination ▸ Adults who lack a risk factor but want protection

12. The number of doses recommended is determined by the presence of specific risk factors (see Table 4).
13. Dose of *Engerix-B* for hemodialysis is 2 mL given at 0, 1, 2, and 6 months. *Recombivax HB* has a separate dialysis formulation (40 mcg in 1 mL) given at 0, 1, and 6 months. This dosing schedule can also be considered for immunocompromised persons.
14. A 4-dose schedule at 0, 1, 2, and 12 months is also FDA-approved.
15. Alternative vaccination schedules (0, 1, and 4 months or 0, 2, and 4 months) are also recommended by ACIP. The minimum interval between doses 1 and 2 is 4 weeks, between doses 2 and 3 is 8 weeks, and between doses 1 and 3 is 16 weeks.

Usual Dose/Schedule	Cost[2]
0.5 mL IM/1 dose	$249.00
0.5 mL IM/1 dose	216.00
0.5 mL IM or SC/1-3 doses[12]	117.10
1 mL IM/2 doses (0 and 6-12 mos)	76.70
1 mL IM/2 doses (0 and 6-18 mos)	74.50
0.5 mL IM/2 doses (0 and 1 mo)	134.20
1 mL IM/3 doses (0, 1, and 6 mos)[13-15]	64.30
1 mL IM/3 doses (0, 1, and 6 mos)[13,15]	62.30[16]
1 mL IM/3 doses (0, 1, and 6 mos)	64.80
1 mL IM/3 doses (0, 1, and 6 mos)[17]	116.80

16. Approximate WAC for 1 dose. WAC = wholesaler acquisition cost or manufacturer's published price to wholesalers; WAC represents a published catalogue or list price and may not represent an actual transactional price. Source: AnalySource® Monthly. July 5, 2022. Reprinted with permission by First Databank, Inc. All rights reserved. ©2022. www.fdbhealth.com/policies/drug-pricing-policy.
17. The minimum interval between doses 1 and 2 is 4 weeks and between doses 2 and 3 is 5 months. A 4-dose accelerated schedule at 0, 7, 21-30 days, and 12 months is also FDA-approved.

Continued on next page

Adult Immunization

Table 1. Some Vaccines for Adults (continued)	
Vaccines	**Recommendations[1]**
Meningococcal	
Serogroups ACWY (MenACWY) Menveo (GSK)[3] MenQuadfi (Sanofi)[3]	▸ Previously unvaccinated adults with specific risk factors[18] ▸ Revaccination every 5 years for those previously vaccinated who remain at high risk
Serogroup B (MenB) Bexsero (GSK)[3,20] Trumenba (Pfizer)[3,20]	▸ Adults with specific risk factors[21]; may administer to persons 16-23 years old (preferred age 16-18 years) not at increased risk ▸ Booster dose of the same vaccine 1 year after completing primary series and every 2-3 years for those at increased risk
Haemophilus influenzae type b (Hib)	
ActHIB (Sanofi)[3] PedvaxHIB (Merck)[3] Hiberix (GSK)[3]	▸ Only for a small number of previously unvaccinated adults with specific risk factors[23]

18. HIV infection, functional or anatomic asplenia, or persistent complement component deficiencies (including impairment induced by eculizumab *[Soliris]* or ravulizumab *[Ultomiris]*).
19. Two doses given ≥8 weeks apart are recommended for adults with asplenia, HIV infection, persistent complement component deficiencies, or eculizumab *(Soliris)* or ravulizumab *(Ultomiris)* use. One dose is recommended for those with other specific risk factors.
20. *Bexsero* and *Trumenba* are not interchangeable.
21. Functional or anatomic asplenia, persons with persistent complement component deficiency or eculizumab or ravulizumab use, those who are at risk from a meningococcal outbreak attributed to serogroup B, and microbiologists routinely exposed to *N. meningitidis*.

Recommendations – Persons born in the US before 1980 are considered immune to varicella, except for healthcare workers and pregnant women, who should be evaluated for evidence of immunity. Evidence of immunity to varicella is demonstrated by a history of varicella or herpes zoster diagnosed or verified by a healthcare provider, laboratory evidence of immunity (not always detected in vaccinated persons), or documentation of vaccination. Adult immigrants who have arrived in the US from tropical countries may be susceptible to varicella. All adults without evidence of immunity should receive 2 doses of the vaccine at least 4 weeks apart.

Usual Dose/Schedule	Cost[2]
0.5 mL IM/1-2 doses[19]	$144.20
0.5 mL IM/1-2 doses[19]	148.70
0.5 mL IM/2 doses (≥1 mo apart)	201.30
0.5 mL IM/2 or 3 doses[22]	168.20
0.5 mL IM/1 or 3 doses[23]	18.20
	28.10
	12.00

22. Healthy young adults 16-23 years old not at increased risk for meningococcal disease may receive a 2-dose series (0 and 6 months). Those with specific risk factors should receive a 3-dose series (0, 1-2, and 6 months).

23. One dose for unimmunized asplenic persons and those undergoing elective splenectomy. Three doses (at least 4 weeks apart) for all recipients of hematopoietic stem cell transplants (beginning 6-12 months after transplant), even if previously vaccinated.

Nonimmune **pregnant women** should receive the first dose postpartum before discharge from the healthcare facility.[11] Immunity after vaccination is probably permanent in the majority of vaccinees.

Adverse Effects – Injection-site reactions such as soreness, erythema, and swelling are common in adults. Other adverse effects include fever and varicella-like rash (at the injection site or generalized, usually occurring within 2-3 weeks after vaccination). Spread of vaccine virus from healthy vaccinees who develop a varicella-like rash to susceptible contacts is rare.

Recipients who have a vaccine-related rash should avoid contact with susceptible individuals who are at high risk of varicella complications, such as immunocompromised persons, pregnant women, and neonates born to nonimmune mothers.

Contraindications – Because it is a live vaccine, varicella vaccine is contraindicated in **pregnant women** and in persons with severe immunodeficiency. It should not be given to persons with a history of anaphylaxis caused by neomycin or gelatin.

ZOSTER — Following resolution of a primary infection, varicella-zoster virus (VZV) persists in a latent form in sensory ganglia. When VZV-specific cell mediated immunity declines, latent VZV can reactivate and cause herpes zoster ("shingles"). About 1 million cases of shingles occur in the US every year.

Shingrix, an adjuvanted recombinant subunit vaccine (RZV), is the only zoster vaccine currently available in the US.[12] *Zostavax,* a live-attenuated vaccine, was withdrawn from the market in 2020.

In observer-blinded clinical trials in >27,000 persons ≥50 years old, RZV was highly effective in preventing herpes zoster (97% in those 50-59 and 60-69 years old and 91% in those 70-79 and ≥80 years old). The duration of protection with RZV is unknown; in persons ≥70 years old, vaccine efficacy was 85.1% in the fourth year after vaccination.[13,14] In 2021, the FDA expanded the indication for use of RZV to include adults ≥18 years old who are or will be at elevated risk of herpes zoster because of disease- or therapy-induced immunodeficiency or immunosuppression. In a trial in 1846 immunocompromised adults who had received an autologous hematopoietic stem cell transplant, and in a post-hoc analysis of a similar trial in 569 adults who were receiving immunosuppressive therapy for hematologic malignancies, RZV significantly decreased the incidence of herpes zoster occurring ≥1 month after the second dose by 68% and 87%, respectively, compared to placebo.[15]

Recommendations – Immunocompetent adults ≥50 years old, including those with a history of herpes zoster and those who have already received the live-attenuated vaccine, and adults ≥19 years old who are or will be immunodeficient or immunosuppressed because of disease or therapy should be vaccinated with two doses of RZV (2-6 months apart). Immunocompromised patients who would benefit from a shorter vaccination schedule can be given the second dose 1-2 months after the first.[15-17]

Adverse Effects – Common adverse effects of RZV include myalgia (45%), fatigue (45%), headache (38%), shivering (27%), fever (21%), GI symptoms (17%), and injection-site pain (78%), redness (38%) and swelling (26%). The adverse effects of RZV in immunocompromised persons appear to be comparable to those in healthy older adults. Use of RZV in adults ≥65 years old has been associated with an increased risk of Guillain-Barré syndrome in the 6 weeks after vaccination.[18]

Unlike the previously available live vaccine, RZV is not contraindicated in **pregnant women**, but its safety and efficacy in this population has not yet been established.

HUMAN PAPILLOMAVIRUS (HPV) — Most HPV infections clear spontaneously without clinical sequelae, but persistent infection with an oncogenic HPV type can cause abnormalities that may progress to cancer. HPV vaccination has resulted in significant declines in the prevalence of vaccine-type HPV infections, anogenital warts, and cervical precancers.[19] However, the incidence of HPV infection and HPV-related cancer is rising in men.[20]

A recombinant 9-valent vaccine (9vHPV; *Gardasil 9*) is the only HPV vaccine available in the US. It is licensed by the FDA for use in both men and women 9 through 45 years old to prevent diseases associated with HPV types 6, 11, 16, 18, 31, 33, 45, 52, and 58, including genital warts and cervical, vulvar, vaginal, and anal precancerous lesions and

Table 2. Some Adverse Effects of Vaccines

Tetanus, Diphtheria, and Pertussis

- Injection-site reactions (usually mild)
- Fever and injection-site pain more common with Tdap than with Td
- Arthus-type reactions after repeated vaccinations (rare)

Measles, Mumps, and Rubella

- Injection-site pain, fever, rash, and transient arthralgias
- Anaphylactic reactions and thrombocytopenic purpura (rare)
- Contraindicated in those with a history of allergic reaction to neomycin (*M-M-R II* or *Priorix*) or gelatin (*M-M-R II*)

Varicella

- Injection-site soreness, erythema, swelling, fever
- Varicella-like rash (at injection site or generalized) 2-3 weeks after vaccination; can rarely result in spread of vaccine virus to susceptible contacts
- Contraindicated in persons with a history of anaphylaxis caused by neomycin or gelatin

Zoster

- Injection-site pain, redness, and swelling, myalgia, fatigue, headache, shivering, fever, and GI symptoms are common
- Increased risk of Guillain-Barré syndrome in adults ≥65 years old in the 6 weeks after vaccination

Human Papillomavirus

- Injection-site pain, swelling, erythema
- Syncope; patients should be seated or lying down during administration and observed for 15 minutes afterwards

Pneumococcal

- Injection-site pain and swelling, myalgia, headache, fatigue, and arthralgia
- PCV13, PCV15, and PCV20 contraindicated in persons with severe allergy to diphtheria toxoid

Hepatitis A

- Injection-site pain, swelling, erythema
- Mild systemic reactions (e.g., malaise, low-grade fever, fatigue) in <10%

Hepatitis B

- Injection-site pain, erythema and swelling; more common with *Heplisav-B* and *PreHevbrio* than with *Engerix-B*

Continued on next page

Table 2. Some Adverse Effects of Vaccines (continued)
Meningococcal (MenACWY and MenB)
► Injection-site pain, erythema, and induration, headache, myalgia, and malaise
Haemophilus Influenzae Type B
► Not studied in adults
► In children: injection-site erythema, pain and swelling, mild fever, irritability, vomiting, and diarrhea
► Monovalent vaccines contraindicated in those with a history of severe allergic reaction to dry natural latex

cancer.[21] It is also indicated for prevention of HPV-related oropharyngeal and other head and neck cancers, but clinical data are lacking.

Recommendations – Routine HPV vaccination is recommended for girls and boys 11-12 years old (can start at age 9). Catch-up HPV vaccination is recommended for all persons through age 26 years who are not adequately vaccinated and may be considered for some persons 27-45 years old who might be at risk for acquiring new HPV infections, such as those who have a new sex partner. Previously unvaccinated persons 15 through 26 years old should receive a 3-dose series (0, 1-2, and 6 months); a 2-dose schedule (0 and 6-12 months) is recommended for those who start the series before age 15 years. Adults who received 1 dose or 2 doses <5 months apart before age 15 years should receive 1 additional dose. Immuno-compromised persons are at higher risk for HPV infection and should be vaccinated with a 3-dose series.[19]

Although vaccination should ideally be completed before the onset of sexual activity, persons ≤26 years old who have already been exposed to HPV or diagnosed with HPV infection (based on an abnormal Pap smear or presence of genital warts) should also be vaccinated because they may not have been exposed to all the HPV types included in the vaccine. A schedule started with the previously available bivalent or quadriva-lent vaccine *(Cervarix; Gardasil)* can be completed with 9vHPV. The

Table 3. Adult Vaccines for Special Populations*

Risk Groups	HPV	Td/Tdap	Influenza	Pneumo-coccal
Pregnancy	NR[1]	✓[2]	✓[3]	NR[4]
Immunocompromising conditions[8,9] (except HIV)	✓	✓	✓[3]	✓[10]
Diabetes	✓	✓	✓[16]	✓[10]
Cardiac or pulmonary[18] disease, or chronic alcoholism	✓	✓	✓[16]	✓[10]
Asplenia,[19] complement deficiencies (including eculizumab or ravulizumab use)	✓	✓	✓[3,20]	✓[10]
End-stage kidney disease (including hemodialysis)	✓	✓	✓[16]	✓[10]
Chronic liver disease	✓	✓	✓[16]	✓[10]
HIV[6]				
CD4 count <200 cells/mcL	✓	✓	✓[3]	✓[10]
CD4 count ≥200 cells/mcL	✓	✓	✓[3]	✓[10]
Healthcare workers	✓	✓	✓	RF[10]
Men who have sex with men	✓	✓	✓	RF[10]

*See Table 1 for age restrictions

✓ = recommended; RF = recommended if another risk factor is present; X = contraindicated; NR = no recommendation; RZV = recombinant zoster vaccine.

1. Vaccinate after pregnancy.
2. Women should receive Tdap during each pregnancy, preferably during the early part of gestational weeks 27 through 36.
3. Only inactivated influenza vaccine is recommended.
4. For PCV15 or PCV20, no data are available. For PPSV23, insufficient data for specific recommendation; no adverse effects have been reported in newborns whose mothers were vaccinated during pregnancy.
5. Pregnant women who are not immune to rubella and/or varicella should receive one dose of MMR vaccine and/or varicella vaccine after delivery and before discharge from the healthcare facility. The second dose of varicella should be given 4-8 weeks after the first dose.
6. Only *Engerix-B, Recombivax B* or *Twinrix* are recommended.
7. MenACWY may be used if otherwise indicated. For MenB, base decision on risk vs benefit.
8. See also published guidelines for vaccination of immunocompromised hosts (LG Rubin et al. Clin Infect Dis 2014; 58:e44; M Tomblyn et al. Biol Blood Marrow Transplant 2009; 15:1143).
9. If possible, indicated vaccines should be given before starting chemotherapy, treatment with other immunosuppressive drugs, or radiation.
10. PCV20 or PCV15 followed by PPSV23 recommended for all patients ≥65 years old and for those ≥19 years old with risk factors (see Table 4).
11. Persons with leukemia, lymphoma, or other malignancies in remission with no recent history (≥3 months) of chemotherapy are not considered severely immunosuppressed for the purpose of receiving live-virus vaccines.
12. Wait at least 1 month after discontinuing long-term administration of high-dose corticosteroids before giving a live-virus vaccine. The definition of high-dose or long-term corticosteroids is considered by most clinicians to be ≥20 mg/day of prednisone or its equivalent for ≥14 days. Short-term (<2 weeks) treatment, low to moderate doses, long-term alternate-day treatment with short-acting preparations, maintenance physiologic doses (replacement therapy), or steroids administered topically, by aerosol, or by intra-articular, bursal, or tendon injection are not considered contraindications to live-virus vaccines.

MMR	Vari-cella	Zoster (RZV)	Hep B	Hep A	Meningo-coccal	Hib
X[5]	X[5]	NR	✓[6]	RF	RF[7]	NR
X[11,12]	X[11,12]	✓[13]	✓[14]	RF	RF	✓[15]
✓	✓	✓[13]	✓[17]	RF	RF	RF
✓	✓	✓[13]	✓[14]	RF	RF	RF
✓	✓	✓[13]	✓[14]	RF	✓	✓[21]
✓	✓	✓[13]	✓[22]	RF	RF	RF
✓	✓	✓[13]	✓	✓	RF	RF
X	X	✓[13]	✓	✓	✓[24]	RF
✓	✓[23]	✓[13]	✓	✓	✓[24]	RF
✓	✓	✓[13]	✓	RF	RF	RF
✓	✓	✓[13]	✓	RF	RF	RF

13. Recommended for adults ≥50 years old and immunocompromised adults ≥19 years old.
14. Recommended for all adults ≤59 years old and for those ≥60 years old with risk factors (see Table 6).
15. Recommended for hematopoietic stem cell transplant recipients only.
16. Inactivated influenza vaccine is recommended. The live-attenuated vaccine may be used if benefit of protection outweighs risk of adverse reactions.
17. Recommended for adults 19-59 years old, and for those ≥60 years old at the discretion of the treating clinician.
18. Chronic pulmonary diseases include chronic pneumonitis, chronic obstructive pulmonary disease, chronic bronchitis, or asthma.
19. Functional or anatomic asplenia, including elective splenectomy. When possible, persons undergoing elective splenectomy should receive the indicated vaccines ≥2 weeks before surgery.
20. No data exist on the risk for severe or complicated influenza in persons with asplenia. However, influenza is a risk factor for secondary bacterial infections that can be life-threatening in asplenic patients.
21. Only recommended for those who never received a primary series and a booster dose at age ≥12 months or at least 1 dose after the age of 14 months.
22. For adults on hemodialysis the dosage of *Engerix-B* is 2 mL given at 0, 1, 2, and 6 months, and the dosage of *Recombivax HB* is 40 mcg/1 mL (dialysis formulation) given at 0, 1, and 6 months. No dosage has been defined for *Heplisav-B*.
23. Vaccination may be considered (2 doses 3 months apart).
24. MenACWY is recommended. MenB is only recommended for those with other indications.

duration of immunity is not known, but it appears to be at least 8-10 years; booster doses are not currently recommended.

HPV vaccine is not recommended for **pregnant women** due to limited data; no increase in adverse outcomes has been reported among women exposed to 9vHPV during the periconceptional period or during pregnancy.

Adverse Effects – Injection-site reactions such as pain, swelling, and erythema can occur. Syncope has been reported; patients should be seated or lying down during vaccine administration and observed for 15 minutes afterwards.

PNEUMOCOCCAL — Adults with certain underlying medical and immunocompromising conditions and those ≥65 years old are at increased risk of developing invasive pneumococcal disease (IPD).

In 2021, the FDA licensed two new pneumococcal conjugate vaccines for use in adults: *Prevnar 20* (PCV20), which contains antigens from 20 serotypes of pneumococcus, and *Vaxneuvance* (PCV15), which contains antigens from 15 serotypes.[22] Two other pneumococcal vaccines have been used in adults, a conjugate vaccine that contains 13 serotypes of pneumococcus (PCV13; *Prevnar 13*) and a 23-valent pneumococcal polysaccharide vaccine (PPSV23; *Pneumovax 23*). PCV20 and PCV15 contain all of the *Streptococcus pneumoniae* antigens included in PCV13 plus 7 (PCV20) or 2 (PCV15) additional antigens, which account for about 30% (PCV20) and 15% (PCV15) of IPD caused by non-PCV13 serotypes in adults at increased risk. PPSV23 contains 19 of the 20 antigens in PCV20 plus 4 additional antigens, which account for about 10% of IPD caused by non-PCV20 serotypes in at-risk adults.[23]

PPSV23 is effective in preventing IPD, but randomized controlled trials and cohort studies in the general population and in those ≥65 years old have not consistently shown that it decreases the incidence of noninvasive pneumococcal pneumonia, and its protective effect appears to wane after 5 years.[24-26]

Table 4. Pneumococcal Vaccination in Adults[1]

Pneumococcal vaccine-naive

≥65 yrs: PCV20 x 1 dose **OR** PCV15 x 1 dose followed by PPSV23 ≥1 yr later[2]
19-64 yrs with risk factors[3]: PCV20 x 1 dose **OR** PCV15 x 1 dose followed by
  PPSV23 ≥1 yr later[2,4]

Previously received PPSV23 but not conjugate vaccine

≥65 yrs or 19-64 yrs with risk factors[3]: PCV20 or PCV15 x 1 dose ≥1 yr after
  PPSV23

Previously received PCV13 but not all recommended doses of PPSV23

≥65 yrs: PPSV23[5] x 1 dose ≥1 yr after PCV13
19-64 yrs with risk factors[3]: PPSV23[5] x 1 dose ≥1 yr[2] after PCV13[6]

1. CDC. Pneumococcal vaccine timing for adults. April 1, 2022. Available at: https://bit.ly/3SjX8Nf. Accessed September 29, 2022.
2. In adults with immunocompromising conditions (see footnote 3), cochlear implant, or CSF leak, PPSV23 may be administered ≥8 weeks later.
3. Includes patients with certain **underlying medical conditions** (alcoholism, CSF leak, chronic heart/liver/lung disease, cigarette smoking, cochlear implant, diabetes) or **immunocompromising conditions** (chronic renal failure, congenital or acquired asplenia or immunodeficiencies, generalized malignancy, HIV infection, Hodgkin disease, iatrogenic immunosuppression, leukemia, lymphoma, multiple myeloma, nephrotic syndrome, sickle cell disease or other hemoglobinopathies, solid organ transplants).
4. No additional doses required at ≥65 years.
5. One dose of PCV20 may be used if PPSV23 is not available. If PCV20 is used, no additional doses of PPSV23 are needed.
6. Additional doses of PPSV23 (≥5 years apart) are recommended for some persons: 1 dose at ≥65 years for those with an underlying medical condition or CSF leak or cochlear implant; 1 dose at <65 years and 1 at ≥65 years for those with immunocompromising conditions.

In double-blind trials in adults who were pneumococcal vaccine-naive, immune responses elicited by PCV20 and PCV15 were noninferior to those elicited by PCV13 for all 13 matched serotypes. Compared to PPSV23, immune responses elicited by PCV20 were noninferior for 6 out of 7 non-PCV13 serotypes.[22]

Recommendations – Previously unvaccinated adults ≥65 years old or 19-64 years old with certain underlying medical conditions or other risk factors should receive a one-time dose of PCV20 or a dose of PCV15 followed by PPSV23 at least one year later.[27]

Specific recommendations for vaccination of adults based on vaccination status, age and risk factors are listed in Table 4.[28] There is no specific recommendation for vaccination of **pregnant women** due to insufficient data with any of these vaccines.

Adverse Effects – Injection-site pain and swelling, myalgia, headache, fatigue, and arthralgia are common with all pneumococcal vaccines. PCV13, PCV15, and PCV20 are contraindicated for use in persons with a severe allergy to diphtheria toxoid.

HEPATITIS A — Outbreaks of hepatitis A virus (HAV) infection continue to occur in adults, particularly among persons using illicit drugs or experiencing homelessness, because of low hepatitis A vaccine (HepA) coverage and high susceptibility to HAV infection.[29] Two inactivated hepatitis A whole-virus vaccines *(Vaqta, Havrix)* are available in the US. A combination hepatitis A and B vaccine (HepA/HepB; *Twinrix*) that contains half the dose of the hepatitis A component in *Havrix* is also available.

Recommendations – HepA vaccination is recommended for adults with certain risk factors (see Table 5).[30] Those who lack a risk factor but want protection should also receive the vaccine. At least one dose of HepA vaccine should be given to persons with risk factors during a community outbreak and to all those with recent exposure to HAV. Vaccination is no longer recommended for persons who receive blood products for clotting disorders.[29] **Pregnant women** at risk for HAV infection or severe outcome from HAV infection should be vaccinated.

HepA vaccination in adults consists of 2 doses separated by at least 6 months. Antibodies reach protective levels 2-4 weeks after the first dose. The combination HepA/HepB vaccine should be given in 3 doses at 0, 1, and 6 months. HepA/HepB vaccine can also be given in an accelerated 4-dose schedule; the first 3 doses are given at 0, 7, and 21-30 days, and the fourth at 12 months. Patients who have received a first dose of one HepA vaccine can be given a different one to complete the series. Booster doses are not recommended for immunocompetent adults who have completed a primary series.

Table 5. Risk Factors for Hepatitis A Infection in Adults[1]
Increased risk:
► Men who have sex with men
► Illegal drug use
► Homelessness
► Occupational risk[2]
► Travelers going to countries with intermediate or high HAV endemicity and close contacts of international adoptees[3] from these countries
► Settings providing services to adults where a high proportion of the clients are at increased risk[4]
Increased risk for severe disease:
► Chronic liver disease
► HIV infection
1. NP Nelson et al. MMWR Morb Mortal Wkly Rep 2020; 69(RR-5):1.
2. Persons who work with HAV-containing material in a research laboratory or with HAV-infected nonhuman primates.
3. During first 60 days after adoptee's arrival.
4. Includes syringe services programs, homeless shelters, group homes, and daycare facilities for the developmentally disabled.

Adverse Effects – Injection-site reactions such as pain, swelling, and erythema occur in about 60% of vaccine recipients. Systemic complaints such as malaise, low-grade fever, and fatigue are generally mild and occur in less than 10% of vaccinees.

HEPATITIS B — Cases of hepatitis B virus (HBV) infection have been increasing in unimmunized adults 30-49 years old.[31] The hepatitis B vaccination rate among adults was about 30% in 2018.[32]

Four hepatitis B vaccines (HepB) that have been available in the US for use in adults contain a single hepatitis B surface antigen (HBsAg): *Engerix-B, Recombivax HB*, *Twinrix* (HepA/HepB vaccine), and *Heplisav-B,* a newer vaccine that uses a synthetic oligonucleotide immunostimulatory adjuvant.[33] The FDA has now licensed *PreHevbrio*, a recombinant, 3-antigen vaccine.[34]

In clinical trials, two doses of *Heplisav-B* were more immunogenic than three doses of *Engerix-B* in adults 18-70 years old.[35] In 2 randomized, double-blind trials in adults (PROTECT and CONSTANT), *PreHevbrio*

Table 6. Risk Factors for Hepatitis B Infection in Adults ≥60 years old[1]
► Sexual exposure[2]
► Percutaneous or mucosal exposure to blood[3]
► Travel to countries with intermediate or high HBV endemicity
► Hepatitis C virus infection or chronic liver disease
► HIV infection
► Incarceration

1. ML Weng et al. MMWR Morb Mortal Wkly Rep 2020; 71:477.
2. Includes sex partners of persons positive for HBsAg, persons with multiple sex partners, persons seeking treatment for a sexually transmitted infection, men who have sex with men.
3. Includes injection drug users, household contacts of persons positive for HBsAg, residents and staff of facilities for persons with developmental disabilities, healthcare personnel with risk for exposure to blood or blood-contaminated body fluids, persons on maintenance dialysis, persons with diabetes (at the discretion of the treating clinician).

was noninferior to *Engerix-B* after 3 doses; in the PROTECT trial, seroprotection rates were significantly higher with *PreHevbrio* than with *Engerix-B* in those ≥45 years old (89.4% vs 73.1%).[36,37]

Recommendations – Hepatitis B vaccination is now recommended for all adults 19-59 years old. In adults ≥60 years old, it is still only recommended for those with a medical, occupational, or behavioral risk for HBV acquisition (see Table 6), but the vaccine should also be offered to patients ≥60 years old without known risk factors.[32,38]

Pregnant women who are at risk for HBV infection should be vaccinated; until more data are available with *Heplisav-B* and *PreHevbrio*, one of the other HepB vaccines should be used.[39]

Primary immunization with *Heplisav-B* consists of 2 doses (0 and 1 month). Primary immunization with the other HepB vaccines usually consists of 3 doses (0, 1, and 6 months). An alternate schedule (0, 1, and 2 months, followed by a fourth dose at 12 months) is FDA-approved for *Engerix-B* and is only intended for use in those who have recently been exposed to the virus and travelers to high-risk areas. HepA/HepB vaccine can also be given in an accelerated schedule (0, 7, and 21-30 days, followed by a fourth dose at 12 months). If possible, the same vaccine should be used for all doses of a HepB series. However, an interrupted HepB series does not have to be restarted if the same vaccine is not available. One or two doses of *Heplisav-B* can be used as part of a 3-dose series started with *Engerix-B*, *Recombivax HB*, or *Twinrix*.[39] Vaccine-induced immunologic memory is excellent; booster doses are not generally recommended for immunocompetent persons who responded to primary immunization as children or adults.[38]

Adverse Effects – The most common adverse effect of hepatitis B vaccination is pain at the injection site; erythema and swelling can also occur. In clinical trials, injection-site reactions were more common with *Heplisav-B* and *PreHevbrio* than with *Engerix-B*.

MENINGOCOCCAL — Meningococcal disease has a case fatality rate of ~15%, and 10%-20% of survivors experience long-term adverse effects such as hearing loss, limb or digit amputations, and neurologic impairment. In recent years, there have been outbreaks of serogroup B disease in college students[40] and of serogroup C disease in men who have sex with men.[41,42]

Two quadrivalent inactivated vaccines against *Neisseria meningitidis* **serogroups A, C, W, and Y** (MenACWY; *Menveo, MenQuadfi*[43]) are available in the US. Both contain meningococcal capsular polysaccharide antigens conjugated to a protein carrier. The antigens in *Menveo* are conjugated to diphtheria toxin-derived carriers, and those in *MenQuadfi* are conjugated to tetanus toxoid protein. Serologic data show a significant decline in serum antibody titers 3-5 years after vaccination. *MenQuadfi* is the only meningococcal vaccine that is indicated for use in persons ≥56 years old.

Two **serogroup B** meningococcal vaccines (MenB; *Trumenba, Bexsero*) are licensed in the US for use in persons 10-25 years old.[44,45] They were approved based on the results of safety and immunogenicity studies. Their comparative efficacy and duration of immunity are unknown.

Recommendations – Routine vaccination with **MenACWY** is recommended for adolescents 11-18 years old, with a first dose at 11-12 years and a booster dose at 16 years. Two doses given at least 8 weeks apart and one booster dose every 5 years are recommended for adults with HIV infection, functional or anatomic asplenia, or persistent complement component deficiencies (including impairment induced by eculizumab *[Soliris]* or ravulizumab *[Ultomiris]*). One dose of vaccine and revaccination every 5 years should be considered for adults who travel to or live in countries where meningococcal disease is hyperendemic or epidemic, persons who are at risk from a meningococcal disease outbreak attributed to serogroup A, C, W, or Y, microbiologists routinely exposed to *N. meningitidis*, military recruits and first-year college students living in dormitories (if they did not receive MenACWY vaccine at age 16 years or older).[46] MenACWY may be used in **pregnant women** if otherwise indicated.

MenB vaccine is recommended for adults with functional or anatomic asplenia, persons with persistent complement component deficiency or eculizumab or ravulizumab use, those who are at risk from a meningococcal outbreak attributed to serogroup B, and microbiologists routinely exposed to *N. meningitidis*. *Bexsero* should be administered in 2 doses at least one month apart; *Trumenba* should be administered in 3 doses at 0, 1-2, and 6 months. MenB vaccine may also be considered for persons 16 through 23 years old (preferably age 16-18 years) who are not at increased risk for serogroup B meningococcal disease; in this setting, *Trumenba* should be given in 2 doses at least 6 months apart and *Bexsero* in 2 doses one month apart.[46] The vaccines are not interchangeable; the same vaccine must be used for all doses. Persons at increased risk should receive a booster dose of the same vaccine 1 year after completing the primary series and every 2-3 years thereafter. During an outbreak, previously vaccinated persons should receive a single booster dose if ≥1 year has passed since completion of the primary series.[47] MenB vaccination should be deferred in **pregnant women** unless the benefits are thought to outweigh the risks.

Adverse Effects – The most common adverse reactions to *Menveo* and *MenQuadfi* are headache, myalgia, malaise, and injection-site pain, redness, and induration; rates are similar to those with tetanus toxoid.

The most common adverse effects of *Bexsero* and *Trumenba* are pain, erythema, and induration at the injection site, fatigue, headache, and myalgia.

***HAEMOPHILUS INFLUENZAE* TYPE B (Hib)** — Hib can cause bacterial meningitis and other invasive diseases. Adults ≥65 years old and those with immunocompromising conditions are at increased risk for invasive Hib disease.[48] Three monovalent Hib conjugate vaccines (*PedvaxHIB*, *ActHIB,* and *Hiberix*) are available in the US.

Recommendations – Hib vaccination is only recommended for immunocompromised adults who are considered at increased risk for invasive Hib disease.[49] A single dose of any Hib conjugate vaccine should be administered to previously unvaccinated adults who have functional or anatomic asplenia or who are scheduled for an elective splenectomy (preferably ≥14 days before the procedure). Some experts suggest administering one dose to these patients regardless of prior vaccination history. Hematopoietic stem cell transplant recipients, including those who had previously been vaccinated, should receive 3 doses of Hib vaccine (given at least 4 weeks apart) beginning 6-12 months after the transplant. Hib vaccination is not recommended for HIV-infected adults.

Adverse Effects – Hib vaccine has not been studied in adults. In children, erythema, pain and swelling at the injection site, mild fever, irritability, vomiting, and diarrhea have occurred. The monovalent vaccines are contraindicated in those with a history of a severe allergic reaction to dry natural latex.

1. N Murthy et al. Advisory Committee on Immunization Practices recommended immunization schedule for adults aged 19 years or older – United States, 2022. MMWR Morb Mortal Wkly Rep 2022; 71:229.
2. COVID-19 vaccine comparison chart (online only). Med Lett Drugs Ther 2021; 63:e1.
3. Influenza vaccine for 2022-2023. Med Lett Drugs Ther 2022; 64:153.
4. Prevention and treatment of monkeypox. Med Lett Drugs Ther 2022; 64:137.
5. Vaccines for travelers. Med Lett Drugs Ther 2018; 60:185.

6. FP Havers et al. Use of tetanus toxoid, reduced diphtheria toxoid, and acellular pertussis vaccines: updated recommendations of the Advisory Committee on Immunization Practices – United States, 2019. MMWR Morb Mortal Wkly Rep 2020; 69:77.

7. VK Phadke et al. Vaccine refusal and measles outbreaks in the US. JAMA 2020; 324:1344.

8. M Marlow et al. Chapter 9: Mumps. In: Manual for the Surveillance of Vaccine-Preventable Diseases. CDC. December 15, 2021. Available at: https://bit.ly/3E1icEc. Accessed September 29, 2022.

9. HQ McLean et al. Prevention of measles, rubella, congenital rubella syndrome, and mumps, 2013: summary recommendations of the Advisory Committee on Immunization Practices (ACIP). MMWR Recomm Rep 2013; 62(RR-4):1.

10. M Marin et al. Recommendation of the Advisory Committee on Immunization Practices for use of a third dose of mumps virus-containing vaccine in persons at increased risk for mumps during an outbreak. MMWR Morb Mortal Wkly Rep 2018; 67:33.

11. M Marin et al. Prevention of varicella: recommendations of the Advisory Committee on Immunization Practices (ACIP). MMWR Recomm Rep 2007; 56(RR-4):1.

12. Shingrix – an adjuvanted, recombinant herpes zoster vaccine. Med Lett Drugs Ther 2017; 59:195.

13. H Lal et al. Efficacy of an adjuvanted herpes zoster subunit vaccine in older adults. N Engl J Med 2015; 372:2087.

14. AL Cunningham et al. Efficacy of the herpes zoster subunit vaccine in adults 70 years of age or older. N Engl J Med 2016; 375:1019.

15. In brief: Shingrix for immunocompromised adults. Med Lett Drugs Ther 2021; 63:129.

16. KL Dooling et al. Recommendations of the Advisory Committee on Immunization Practices for use of herpes zoster vaccines. MMWR Morb Mortal Wkly Rep 2018; 67:103.

17. TC Anderson et al. Use of recombinant zoster vaccine in immunocompromised adults aged ≥19 years: recommendations of the Advisory Committee on Immunization Practices – United States, 2022. MMWR Morb Mortal Wkly Rep 2022; 71:80.

18. FDA Safety Communication. FDA requires a warning about Guillain-Barré Syndrome (GBS) be included in the prescribing information for Shingrix. March 24, 2021. Available at: https://bit.ly/3lmyvC6. Accessed September 29, 2022.

19. E Meites et al. Human papillomavirus vaccination for adults: updated recommendations of the Advisory Committee on Immunization Practices. MMWR Morb Mortal Wkly Rep 2019; 68:698.

20. JE Tota et al. Anogenital human papillomavirus (HPV) infection, seroprevalence, and risk factors for HPV seropositivity among sexually active men enrolled in a global HPV vaccine trial. Clin Infect Dis 2022; 74:1247.

21. Gardasil 9 – a broader HPV vaccine. Med Lett Drugs Ther 2015; 57:47.

22. Two new pneumococcal vaccines – Prevnar 20 and Vaxneuvance. Med Lett Drugs Ther 2021; 63:188.

23. M Kobayashi. Considerations for age-based and risk-based use of PCV15 and PCV20 among U.S. adults and proposed policy options. ACIP Meeting. October 20, 2021. Available at: https://bit. Ly/2YhkaOi. Accessed September 29, 2022.

24. G Falkenhorst et al. Effectiveness of the 23-valent pneumococcal polysaccharide vaccine (PPV23) against pneumococcal disease in the elderly: systematic review and meta-analysis. PLoS One 2017; 12:e0169368.

25. O Ochoa-Gondar et al. Effectiveness of the 23-valent pneumococcal polysaccharide vaccine against community-acquired pneumonia in the general population age ≥60 years: 3 years of follow-up in the CAPAMIS study. Clin Infect Dis 2014; 58:909.

26. M Suzuki et al. Serotype-specific effectiveness of 23-valent pneumococcal polysaccharide vaccine against pneumococcal pneumonia in adults aged 65 years or older: a multicentre, prospective, test-negative design study. Lancet Infect Dis 2017; 17:313.

27. M Kobayashi et al. Use of 15-valent pneumococcal conjugate vaccine and 20-valent pneumococcal conjugate vaccine among U.S. adults: updated recommendations of the Advisory Committee on Immunization Practices – United States, 2022. MMWR Morb Mortal Wkly Rep 2022; 71:109.

28. CDC. Pneumococcal vaccine timing for adults. April 1, 2022. Available at: https://bit.ly/3SjX8Nf. Accessed September 29, 2022.

29. NP Nelson et al. Prevention of hepatitis A virus infection in the United States: recommendations of the Advisory Committee on Immunization Practices, 2020. MMWR Recomm Rep 2020; 69(RR-5):1.

30. M Doshani et al. Recommendations of the Advisory Committee on Immunization Practices for use of hepatitis A vaccine for persons experiencing homelessness. MMWR Morb Mortal Wkly Rep 2019; 68:153.

31. CDC. Viral hepatitis surveillance report – United States, 2019. May 19, 2021. Available at: https://bit.ly/3BV6V5p. Accessed September 29, 2022.

32. MK Weng et al. Universal hepatitis B vaccination in adults aged 19-59 years: updated recommendations of the Advisory Committee on Immunization Practices – United States, 2022. MMWR Morb Mortal Wkly Rep 2022; 71:477.

33. A two-dose hepatitis B vaccine for adults (Heplisav-B). Med Lett Drugs Ther 2018; 60:17.

34. A three-antigen hepatitis B vaccine (PreHevbrio). Med Lett Drugs Ther 2022; 64:73.

35. S Jackson et al. Immunogenicity of a two-dose investigational hepatitis B vaccine, HBsAg-1018, using a toll-like receptor 9 agonist adjuvant compared with a licensed hepatitis B vaccine in adults. Vaccine 2018; 36:668.

36. T Vesikari et al. Immunogenicity and safety of a tri-antigenic versus a mono-antigenic hepatitis B vaccine in adults (PROTECT): a randomised, double-blind, phase 3 trial. Lancet Infect Dis 2021; 21:1271.

37. T Vesikari et al. Immunogenicity and safety of a 3-antigen hepatitis B vaccine vs a single-antigen hepatitis B vaccine: a phase 3 randomized clinical trial. JAMA Netw Open 2021; 4:e2128652.

38. S Schillie et al. Prevention of hepatitis B virus infection in the United States: recommendations of the Advisory Committee on Immunization Practices. MMWR Recomm Rep 2018; 67(RR-1):1.

39. S Schillie et al. Recommendations of the Advisory Committee on Immunization Practices for use of a hepatitis B vaccine with a novel adjuvant. MMWR Morb Mortal Wkly Rep 2018; 67:455.

40. HM Soeters et al. University-based outbreaks of meningococcal disease cause by serogroup B, United States, 2013-2018. Emerg Infect Dis 2019; 25:434.

41. CH Bozio et al. Meningococcal disease surveillance in men who have sex with men – United States, 2015-2016. MMWR Morb Mortal Wkly Rep 2018; 67:1060.

42. CDC. Meningococcal disease outbreak among gay, bisexual men in Florida 2021-22. August 8, 2022. Available at: https://bit.ly/3rkuFLm. Accessed September 29, 2022.
43. MenQuadfi – a new meningococcal (A, C, W, and Y) vaccine. Med Lett Drugs Ther 2021; 63:78.
44. Bexsero – a second serogroup B meningococcal vaccine. Med Lett Drugs Ther 2015; 57:158.
45. Trumenba: a serogroup B meningococcal vaccine. Med Lett Drugs Ther 2015; 57:5.
46. SA Mbaeyi et al. Meningococcal vaccination: recommendations of the Advisory Committee on Immunization Practices, United States, 2020. MMWR Recomm Rep 2020; 69:1.
47. In brief: New meningococcal serogroup B vaccination recommendations. Med Lett Drugs Ther 2020; 62:191.
48. HM Soeters et al. Current epidemiology and trends in invasive Haemophilus influenzae disease–United States, 2009-2015. Clin Infect Dis 2018; 67:881.
49. EC Briere et al. Prevention and control of Haemophilus influenzae type b disease: recommendations of the Advisory Committee on Immunization Practices (ACIP). MMWR Recomm Rep 2014; 63(RR-1):1.

DRUGS FOR
Benign Prostatic Hyperplasia

Original publication date – May 2022

About 60% of men $\geq$60 years old have clinically relevant prostatic enlargement due to benign prostatic hyperplasia (BPH).[1] The goals of treatment are to decrease lower urinary tract symptoms and to prevent disease progression and complications such as acute urinary retention. The American Urologic Association's guidelines for treatment of BPH were recently updated.[2]

GENERAL APPROACH — Mild BPH symptoms should generally be managed with watchful waiting, nonpharmacologic interventions, and avoidance of drugs that precipitate symptoms, such as oral decongestants and first-generation antihistamines. Patients should be monitored every 6-12 months for changes in symptom severity, urinary flow and retention rates, and prostate size.[3] In patients with moderately to severely bothersome BPH, pharmacotherapy should be added to decrease symptoms and the need for surgical intervention. Surgery is recommended for patients with kidney dysfunction or gross hematuria due to BPH, and in those with recurrent urinary tract infections or bladder stones.[2]

NONPHARMACOLOGIC MANAGEMENT — Lifestyle modifications that can decrease BPH symptoms include fluid restriction and frequent emptying of the bladder (especially just before sleep, travel, or exercise), use of timed voiding and double voiding techniques, performing Kegel exercises during periods of urgency, pelvic floor muscle training,

---

Key Points: Treatment of BPH

► Lifestyle modifications, such as fluid restriction, frequent bladder emptying, and avoidance of bladder irritants, are recommended for patients with BPH of any severity.

► Mildly symptomatic BPH should be managed with watchful waiting; patients should be monitored every 6-12 months. Patients with moderately to severely bothersome BPH should receive pharmacotherapy to decrease symptoms and the need for surgery.

► **Alpha-1 adrenergic antagonists** (alpha blockers) are recommended for patients with moderately to severely symptomatic BPH. They can rapidly relieve symptoms, but they do not slow disease progression.

► The **5α-reductase inhibitors** finasteride and dutasteride can reduce prostatic volume and decrease urinary retention and the need for surgery. They are recommended for use alone or in combination with an alpha blocker in men with prostatic enlargement and moderate to severe BPH symptoms.

► The **phosphodiesterase type 5 inhibitor** tadalafil can decrease BPH symptoms. It may be a useful option for men with comorbid erectile dysfunction and others who want to mitigate the sexual adverse effects of other drugs for BPH.

► An **anticholinergic drug** or a **beta-3 adrenergic agonist** can be added to an alpha blocker to decrease BPH symptoms associated with storage (urgency, frequency, nocturia) and bladder irritation.

► Patients with acute urinary retention should receive at least 3 days of treatment with an alpha blocker before undergoing an initial trial without a catheter.

---

weight loss, limiting consumption of diuretics such as caffeine and alcohol, and avoiding bladder irritants such as heavily seasoned or very spicy or acidic foods or carbonated beverages.[4,5]

ALPHA BLOCKERS — Alpha-1 adrenergic antagonists (alpha blockers) cause relaxation of smooth muscle in the prostate and bladder neck, improving urinary flow. They can decrease the risk of acute urinary retention, but they do not decrease prostate size or slow disease progression. Alpha blockers are recommended for patients with moderately to severely bothersome BPH; they are usually effective within days of starting treatment.

Five alpha blockers are FDA-approved for treatment of BPH. Alfuzosin, doxazosin, and terazosin are nonselective alpha-1 adrenergic antagonists. Tamsulosin and silodosin are selective for the prostatic alpha-1A receptor. Nonselective and selective drugs are generally considered similar in efficacy.[6]

Adverse Effects – The most significant adverse effects associated with alpha blockers are dizziness, hypotension, and ejaculative dysfunction (anejaculation or retrograde ejaculation). Doxazosin and terazosin are most likely to cause hypotension[7]; they should be titrated slowly to reduce the risk of orthostasis and syncope. Tamsulosin and silodosin are more likely than the nonselective alpha blockers to cause ejaculative dysfunction.[8]

Use of alpha blockers in patients undergoing cataract surgery has been associated with an increased risk of intraoperative floppy iris syndrome; the risk appears to be greatest with tamsulosin.[9] Withholding tamsulosin in the days before cataract surgery can decrease but not eliminate the risk.[10] In patients who are scheduled to undergo cataract surgery, alpha blocker therapy should not be started until after completion of the procedure.

Drug and Genome Interactions – Use of alpha blockers with phosphodiesterase type 5 (PDE-5) inhibitors or other drugs that lower blood pressure can result in additive effects.

Alfuzosin, doxazosin, silodosin, and tamsulosin are metabolized by CYP3A4; coadministration of CYP3A4 inhibitors can increase their serum concentrations. Alfuzosin and silodosin are contraindicated for use with CYP3A4 inhibitors. Tamsulosin is also metabolized by CYP2D6; use with a CYP2D6 inhibitor (e.g., darifenacin, mirabegron) or in patients who are CYP2D6 poor metabolizers can increase tamsulosin serum concentrations. Silodosin is transported by P-glycoprotein (P-gp); use with P-gp inhibitors also can increase its serum concentrations and the risk of toxicity.[11]

5α-REDUCTASE INHIBITORS — The 5α-reductase inhibitors finasteride and dutasteride block prostatic conversion of testosterone to dihydrotestosterone, decreasing the size of the prostate over several months

Table 1. Some Drugs for Benign Prostatic Hyperplasia

Drug	Some Formulations
Alpha-1 Adrenergic Antagonists	
Alfuzosin – generic *Uroxatral* (Concordia)	10 mg ER tabs
Doxazosin – generic *Cardura* (Pfizer)	1, 2, 4, 8 mg tabs
extended-release – *Cardura XL*	4, 8 mg ER tabs
Terazosin – generic	1, 2, 5, 10 mg caps
Silodosin[7] – generic *Rapaflo* (Allergan)	4, 8 mg caps
Tamsulosin[7] – generic *Flomax* (Sanofi)	0.4 mg caps
5α-Reductase Inhibitors	
Dutasteride – generic *Avodart* (Woodward)	0.5 mg caps
Finasteride – generic *Proscar* (MSD)	5 mg tabs
5α-Reductase Inhibitor/Alpha-1 Adrenergic Antagonist Combination	
Dutasteride/tamsulosin – generic *Jalyn* (Woodward)	0.5/0.4 mg ER caps
Phosphodiesterase-5 Inhibitor	
Tadalafil – generic *Cialis* (Lilly)	5 mg tabs
5α-Reductase Inhibitor/Phosphodiesterase-5 Inhibitor Combination	
Finasteride/tadalafil – *Entadfi* (Veru)	5/5 mg tabs

ER = extended-release
1. Approximate WAC for a 30-day supply at the lowest usual maintenance dosage. WAC = wholesaler acquisition cost or manufacturer's published price to wholesalers; WAC represents a published catalogue or list price and may not represent an actual transactional price. Source: AnalySource® Monthly. April 5, 2022. Reprinted with permission by First Databank, Inc. All rights reserved. ©2022. www.fdbhealth.com/drug-pricing-policy.
2. Taken with the same meal each day.
3. The daily dose can be doubled every 1-2 weeks to a maximum of 8 mg based on response and tolerability.
4. The daily dose can be increased to 8 mg after 3-4 weeks based on response and tolerability.

Usual Initial Dosage	Usual Maintenance Dosage	Cost[1]
10 mg PO once/day[2]	10 mg PO once/day[2]	$10.30
		768.00
1 mg PO once/day[3]	1-8 mg PO once/day	14.10
		161.30
4 mg PO qAM[4,5]	4-8 mg PO qAM[4,5]	194.70
1 mg PO qhs[6]	10-20 mg PO qhs	13.90
8 mg PO once/day[8]	8 mg PO once/day[8]	35.00
		261.50
0.4 mg PO once/day	0.4-0.8 mg PO once/day	9.00
		277.90
0.5 mg PO once/day	0.5 mg PO once/day	14.90
		277.90
5 mg PO once/day	5 mg PO once/day	12.00
		141.30
0.5/0.4 mg PO once/day[9]	0.5/0.4 mg PO once/day[9]	129.40
		227.90
5 mg PO once/day	5 mg PO once/day	17.20
		355.80
5/5 mg PO once/day	5/5 mg PO once/day[10]	95.10

5. Taken with breakfast.
6. The daily dose should be increased sequentially to 2 mg, 5 mg, and then 10 mg based on clinical response.
7. Selective for the prostatic alpha-1A receptor.
8. Taken with a meal. In patients with moderate renal impairment (CrCl 30-50 mL/min), the recommended dosage is 4 mg once/day. Contraindicated for use in patients with severe renal impairment (CrCl <30 mL/min) or severe hepatic impairment (Child-Pugh C). Capsules may be swallowed whole, or their contents may sprinkled over applesauce and consumed immediately with 8 oz of cool water.
9. Taken 30 minutes after the same meal each day.
10. Taken for up to 26 weeks.

Continued on next page

Table 1. Some Drugs for Benign Prostatic Hyperplasia (continued)	
Drug	**Some Formulations**
Anticholinergic Drugs[11]	
Darifenacin – generic	7.5, 15 mg ER tabs
Fesoterodine – *Toviaz* (Pfizer)	4, 8 mg ER tabs
Oxybutynin – generic extended-release – generic *Ditropan XL* (Janssen)	5 mg tabs 5, 10, 15 mg ER tabs
Solifenacin – generic *Vesicare* (Astellas)	5, 10 mg tabs

Tolterodine – generic
  Detrol (Pfizer)
extended-release – generic
  Detrol LA
	1, 2 mg tabs
	
	2, 4 mg ER caps

Trospium – generic extended-release – generic	20 mg tabs 60 mg ER caps
Beta-3 Adrenergic Agonists[11]	
Mirabegron – *Myrbetriq* (Astellas)	25, 50 mg ER tabs
Vibegron – *Gemtesa* (Urovant)	75 mg tabs

ER = extended-release
11. Not FDA-approved for treatment of benign prostatic hyperplasia.
12. Taken with water.
13. According to the package insert, an initial dosage of 2.5 mg bid-tid can be considered for patients who are frail and elderly.
14. Taken on an empty stomach at least 1 hour before a meal.
15. In patients with severe renal impairment (CrCl <30 mL/min), the recommended dosage is 20 mg once/day. A dosage of 20 mg once/day can also be considered for patients ≥75 years old based on tolerability.

and consequently increasing the rate of urinary flow. Though patients may not experience maximal symptomatic relief for up to 6 months after starting a 5α-reductase inhibitor, the reduction in prostatic volume can decrease urinary retention and the need for surgery.[12] Use of a 5α-reductase inhibitor alone or in combination with an alpha blocker is recommended in men with moderately to severely bothersome BPH and prostatic enlargement.

Adverse Effects – Adverse effects of 5α-reductase inhibitors include sexual dysfunction (e.g., impotence, decreased libido, ejaculation disorder), breast

Usual Initial Dosage	Usual Maintenance Dosage	Cost[1]
7.5 mg PO once/day[12]	7.5-15 mg PO once/day[12]	$105.10
4 mg PO once/day	4-8 mg PO once/day	376.60
5 mg PO bid-tid[13]	5 mg PO bid-qid	16.80
5-10 mg PO once/day	5-30 mg PO once/day	35.80
		190.60
5 mg PO once/day[12]	5-10 mg PO once/day[12]	11.50
		385.50
2 mg PO bid	1-2 mg PO bid	70.00
		450.00
4 mg PO once/day[12]	2-4 mg PO once/day[12]	150.30
		366.80
20 mg PO bid[14,15]	20 mg PO bid[14,15]	36.50
60 mg PO qAM[12,14]	60 mg PO qAM[12,14]	138.60
25 mg PO once/day	25-50 mg PO once/day[16]	429.70
75 mg PO once/day[12,17]	75 mg PO once/day[12,17]	458.40

16. In patients with severe renal impairment (eGFR 15-29 mL/min/1.73 m^2) or moderate hepatic impairment (Child-Pugh B), the maximum daily dose is 25 mg. Not recommended for use in patients with end-stage renal disease (eGFR <15 mL/min/1.73 m^2 or requiring dialysis) or severe hepatic impairment (Child-Pugh C).
17. Tablets can be swallowed whole or crushed and taken with a tablespoon of applesauce.

enlargement or tenderness, and rash.[13,14] Coadministration of the PDE-5 inhibitor tadalafil may mitigate some of the sexual adverse effects associated with 5α-reductase inhibitors.

Both finasteride and dutasteride have been associated with a lower overall incidence of prostate cancer, but a higher incidence of high-grade prostate cancer, compared to placebo.[15,16] Breast cancer has occurred rarely in men taking 5α-reductase inhibitors; a causal relationship has not been established.

In observational studies, 5α-reductase inhibitors have been associated with diabetes, dementia, depression, and suicidality, but data supporting these associations are generally mixed and unconvincing.[17-21]

Drug and Laboratory Interactions – Dutasteride is a substrate of CYP3A4; concomitant use of CYP3A4 inhibitors could increase its serum concentrations.[11]

Use of a 5α-reductase inhibitor decreases serum prostate-specific antigen (PSA) concentrations by about 50%; a new PSA baseline should be established about 6 months after starting treatment. Increases in PSA levels in patients taking a 5α-reductase inhibitor could signal development of prostate cancer even if levels remain within normal limits.

PDE-5 INHIBITOR — The PDE-5 inhibitor tadalafil is FDA-approved for treatment of BPH with or without erectile dysfunction. Inhibition of PDE-5 is thought to decrease smooth muscle tone and proliferation in the prostate, bladder neck, and urethra, leading to improved urination.[22] Tadalafil does not decrease prostate size or slow disease progression. Maximal symptomatic relief usually occurs within about one month of starting the drug.

Used as monotherapy, tadalafil is similar in efficacy to alpha blockers in decreasing BPH symptoms. Adding once-daily tadalafil to an alpha blocker or a 5α-reductase inhibitor may mitigate sexual adverse effects, but a Cochrane review found that such use does not have any clinically significant additive effects on BPH symptoms.[23]

A fixed-dose combination of finasteride and tadalafil (*Entadfi*; both drugs are available generically) is FDA-approved for initial (up to 26 weeks') treatment of BPH in men with an enlarged prostate. In a double-blind trial, the combination decreased BPH symptoms more than finasteride alone in the first weeks of treatment (before finasteride achieved its maximal effect), but by 26 weeks, the difference between the two groups was clinically negligible.[24,25]

Adverse Effects – Adverse effects of tadalafil include headache, dizziness, dyspepsia, back pain, and myalgia. Priapism leading to irreversible erectile tissue damage can occur. Serious ophthalmic adverse effects such as serous retinal detachment, retinal vascular occlusion, and ischemic optic neuropathy can occur rarely with PDE-5 inhibitors.[26] A sudden loss of hearing has also been reported with use of these drugs, but causality has not been established.

Drug Interactions – Tadalafil can potentiate the hypotensive effects of alpha blockers, guanylate cyclase stimulators (riociguat, vericiguat), nitrates, and antihypertensive drugs; concurrent use with a guanylate cyclase stimulator or nitrate is contraindicated. Coadministration of alcohol and tadalafil can cause additive vasodilation leading to orthostasis. Strong CYP3A4 inhibitors such as ketoconazole can increase serum concentrations of tadalafil and concomitant use is not recommended.[11]

ANTICHOLINERGIC DRUGS — Commonly used for treatment of overactive bladder, anticholinergic drugs have also been used off-label either alone or, more typically, in combination with an alpha blocker for treatment of BPH in patients whose symptoms are mainly related to bladder irritation and urine storage (urgency, frequency, nocturia). They have improved quality of life measures in patients with these symptoms,[27-29] but they do not slow disease progression or treat symptoms related to bladder outlet obstruction. Maximal symptomatic relief generally occurs within 1-2 weeks of starting treatment.[22]

Adverse Effects – Common anticholinergic adverse effects include dry mouth, nausea, constipation, and confusion; use of an M_3-selective anticholinergic drug (darifenacin or solifenacin) may decrease the risk of these adverse effects. Long-term use of anticholinergic drugs in older adults has been associated with development of dementia.[30]

Use of anticholinergic drugs for BPH has been associated with urinary retention, but the absolute risk appears to be small when they are combined with alpha blockers.[31] A post-void residual urine measurement should be obtained before starting an anticholinergic drug and periodically during treatment.

Drug Interactions – Coadministration of an anticholinergic drug and a beta-3 adrenergic agonist may increase the risk of urinary retention. Use of anticholinergic drugs with other drugs that have anticholinergic properties (e.g., paroxetine) can result in additive adverse effects. Darifenacin, solifenacin, tolterodine, fesoterodine, and oxybutynin are CYP3A4 substrates; inhibitors of CYP3A4 can increase their serum concentrations. Darifenacin is a moderate CYP2D6 inhibitor; it can increase serum concentrations and adverse effects of drugs that are metabolized by CYP2D6 (e.g., tamsulosin).[11] The antihyperglycemic drug metformin can decrease serum concentrations of trospium.

BETA-3 AGONISTS — The beta-3 adrenergic agonists mirabegron and vibegron are FDA-approved for treatment of overactive bladder,[32,33] but they have also been used off-label in combination with an alpha blocker for treatment of BPH in patients whose symptoms are mainly related to bladder irritation and urine storage (urgency, frequency, nocturia). Activation of beta-3 receptors in the bladder causes relaxation of detrusor smooth muscle during the storage phase of the fill-void cycle and increases bladder capacity. Beta-3 agonists do not slow disease progression or treat symptoms related to bladder outlet obstruction.

In a 12-week open-label trial in men with BPH and persistent overactive bladder symptoms, addition of mirabegron to the alpha blocker silodosin was similar to addition of the anticholinergic drug fesoterodine in improving symptoms and quality of life.[34] Monotherapy with a beta-3 adrenergic agonist has not been shown to improve BPH symptoms compared to placebo.[35]

Adverse Effects – Beta-3 agonists are generally well tolerated; headache, dizziness, nasopharyngitis, and GI upset can occur. Urinary retention has been reported. Mirabegron can increase blood pressure; it is not recommended for use in patients with severe uncontrolled hypertension (SBP

≥180 mm Hg or DBP ≥110 mm Hg). Leukocytoclastic vasculitis has occurred rarely with use of mirabegron.

Drug Interactions – Coadministration of a beta-3 adrenergic agonist and an anticholinergic drug may increase the risk of urinary retention. Mirabegron is a moderate inhibitor of CYP2D6; it can increase the serum concentrations and toxicity of CYP2D6 substrates (e.g., tamsulosin).[11] Vibegron increases serum concentrations of digoxin.

SUPPLEMENTS — Various dietary supplements and herbal products, including saw palmetto (*Serenoa repens* or *Sabal serrulatum*) extract, have been suggested as therapeutic options for management of BPH. There is no convincing evidence that any of these products provide meaningful symptomatic relief or affect disease progression. A Cochrane review of 32 randomized controlled trials concluded that saw palmetto, even at higher-than-usual doses, does not improve BPH symptoms compared to placebo.[36]

ACUTE URINARY RETENTION — Patients with acute urinary retention due to BPH should generally be treated with an alpha blocker if they are not already taking one; alfuzosin and tamsulosin have been studied most extensively for this indication. Patients should complete at least 3 days of treatment with an alpha blocker before undergoing an initial trial without a catheter. Maintenance treatment with an alpha blocker and a 5α-reductase inhibitor can decrease the risk of recurrence.[2,37]

1. KB Egan. The epidemiology of benign prostatic hyperplasia associated with lower urinary tract symptoms: prevalence and incident rates. Urol Clin North Am 2016; 43:289.
2. LB Lerner et al. Management of lower urinary tract symptoms attributed to benign prostatic hyperplasia: AUA guideline part I–initial work-up and medical management. J Urol 2021; 206:806.
3. DK Newman et al. An evidence-based strategy for the conservative management of the male patient with incontinence. Curr Opin Urol 2014; 24:553.
4. CT Brown et al. Self management for men with lower urinary tract symptoms: randomised controlled trial. BMJ 2007; 334:25.
5. KL Burgio et al. Effectiveness of combined behavioral and drug therapy for overactive bladder symptoms in men: a randomized clinical trial. JAMA Intern Med 2020; 180:411.

6. JQ Yuan et al. Comparative effectiveness and safety of monodrug therapies for lower urinary tract symptoms associated with benign prostatic hyperplasia: a network meta-analysis. Medicine (Baltimore) 2015; 94:e974.

7. DA Schwinn et al. alpha1-adrenoceptor subtype selectivity and lower urinary tract symptoms. Mayo Clin Proc 2004; 79:1423.

8. M Gacci et al. Impact of medical treatments for male lower urinary tract symptoms due to benign prostatic hyperplasia on ejaculatory function: a systematic review and meta-analysis. J Sex Med 2014; 11:1554.

9. IP Chatziralli and TN Sergentanis. Risk factors for intraoperative floppy iris syndrome: a meta-analysis. Ophthalmology 2011; 118:730.

10. CM Bell et al. Association between tamsulosin and serious ophthalmic adverse events in older men following cataract surgery. JAMA 2009; 301:1991.

11. Inhibitors and inducers of CYP enzymes, P-glycoprotein, and other transporters. Med Lett Drugs Ther 2021 October 20 (epub). Available at: medicalletter.org/downloads/CYP_PGP_Tables.pdf.

12. JD McConnell et al. The long-term effect of doxazosin, finasteride, and combination therapy on the clinical progression of benign prostatic hyperplasia. N Engl J Med 2003; 349:2387.

13. CW Fwu et al. Change in sexual function in men with lower urinary tract symptoms/benign prostatic hyperplasia associated with long-term treatment with doxazosin, finasteride and combined therapy. J Urol 2014; 191:1828.

14. CG Roehrborn et al. A prospective randomised placebo-controlled study of the impact of dutasteride/tamsulosin combination therapy on sexual function domains in sexually active men with lower urinary tract symptoms (LUTS) secondary to benign prostatic hyperplasia (BPH). BJU Int 2018; 121:647.

15. L Wang et al. Association of finasteride with prostate cancer: a systematic review and meta-analysis. Medicine (Baltimore) 2020; 99:e19486.

16. GL Andriole et al. Effect of dutasteride on the risk of prostate cancer. N Engl J Med 2010; 362:1192.

17. B Welk et al. The risk of dementia with the use of 5 alpha reductase inhibitors. J Neurol Sci 2017; 379:109.

18. B Welk et al. Association of suicidality and depression with 5α-reductase inhibitors. JAMA Intern Med 2017; 177:683.

19. KW Hagberg et al. Risk of incident antidepressant-treated depression associated with use of 5α-reductase inhibitors compared with use of α-Blockers in men with benign prostatic hyperplasia: a population-based study using the Clinical Practice Research Datalink. Pharmacotherapy 2017; 37:517.

20. L Wei et al. Incidence of type 2 diabetes mellitus in men receiving steroid 5α-reductase inhibitors: population based cohort study. BMJ 2019; 365:l1204.

21. SS Lee et al. 5-alpha-reductase inhibitors and the risk of diabetes mellitus: a nationwide population-based study. Prostate 2016; 76:41.

22. S Albisinni et al. New medical treatments for lower urinary tract symptoms due to benign prostatic hyperplasia and future perspectives. BMC Urol 2016; 16:58.

23. S Pattanaik et al. Phosphodiesterase inhibitors for lower urinary tract symptoms consistent with benign prostatic hyperplasia. Cochrane Database Syst Rev 2018; 11:CD010060.

24. A fixed-dose combination of finasteride and tadalafil (Entadfi) for BPH. Med Lett Drugs Ther 2022; 64:e1.

25. A Casabé et al. Efficacy and safety of the coadministration of tadalafil once daily with finasteride for 6 months in men with lower urinary tract symptoms and prostatic enlargement secondary to benign prostatic hyperplasia. J Urol 2014; 191:727.

26. M Etminan et al. Risk of ocular adverse events associated with use of phosphodiesterase 5 inhibitors in men in the US. JAMA Ophthalmol 2022 April 7 (epub).

27. P Van Kerrebroeck et al. Efficacy and safety of solifenacin plus tamsulosin OCAS in men with voiding and storage lower urinary tract symptoms: results from a phase 2, dose-finding study (SATURN). Eur Urol 2013; 64:398.

28. P van Kerrebroeck et al. Combination therapy with solifenacin and tamsulosin oral controlled absorption system in a single tablet for lower urinary tract symptoms in men: efficacy and safety results from the randomised controlled NEPTUNE trial. Eur Urol 2013; 64:1003.

29. SA Kaplan et al. Safety and tolerability of solifenacin add-on therapy to alpha-blocker treated men with residual urgency and frequency. J Urol 2009; 182:2825.

30. CAC Coupland et al. Anticholinergic drug exposure and the risk of dementia: a nested case-control study. JAMA Intern Med 2019; 179:1084.

31. TH Kim et al. Comparison of the efficacy and safety of tolterodine 2 mg and 4 mg combined with an α-blocker in men with lower urinary tract symptoms (LUTS) and overactive bladder: a randomized controlled trial. BJU Int 2016; 117:307.

32. Mirabegron (Myrbetriq) for overactive bladder. Med Lett Drugs Ther 2013; 55:13.

33. Vibegron (Gemtesa) for overactive bladder. Med Lett Drugs Ther 2021; 63:67.

34. Y Matsukawa et al. Comparison in the efficacy of fesoterodine or mirabegron add-on therapy to silodosin for patients with benign prostatic hyperplasia complicated by overactive bladder: a randomized, prospective trial using urodynamic studies. Neurourol Urodyn 2019; 38:941.

35. VW Nitti et al. Urodynamics and safety of the β3-adrenoceptor agonist mirabegron in males with lower urinary tract symptoms and bladder outlet obstruction. J Urol 2013; 190:1320.

36. R MacDonald et al. Serenoa repens monotherapy for benign prostatic hyperplasia (BPH): an updated Cochrane systematic review. BJU Int 2012; 109:1756.

37. P Toren et al. Effect of dutasteride on clinical progression of benign prostatic hyperplasia in asymptomatic men with enlarged prostate: a post hoc analysis of the REDUCE study. BMJ 2013; 346:f2109.

DRUGS FOR
Cognitive Loss and Dementia

Original publication date – August 2022

Alzheimer's disease (AD) is the most common cause of dementia, but cognitive decline is also associated with other neurological conditions such as Parkinson's disease, dementia with Lewy bodies, vascular dementia, and frontotemporal dementia.

Mild cognitive impairment (MCI) is generally defined as cognitive decline that is greater than expected based on an individual's age and level of education, but that does not interfere with activities of daily living; it may be a transitional state between the cognitive changes of normal aging and dementia.[1]

Treatment of reversible dementia due to drug toxicity, infection, or metabolic disorders is not reviewed here.

CHOLINESTERASE INHIBITORS

Cognitive decline in AD is associated with depletion of acetylcholine, which is involved in learning and memory. Acetylcholinesterase inhibitors increase acetylcholine concentrations in the brain and can produce modest improvements in cognition, psychological symptoms, and activities of daily living.[2]

Donepezil, galantamine, and rivastigmine are FDA-approved for treatment of AD dementia based on statistically significant improvements

47

Key Points: Drugs for Cognitive Loss and Dementia

► The acetylcholinesterase inhibitors donepezil, rivastigmine, and galantamine can modestly improve symptoms of dementia in patients with Alzheimer's disease. Transdermal rivastigmine and donepezil may be less likely to cause GI adverse effects than their oral formulations.

► The NMDA-receptor antagonist memantine may provide some modest benefit in patients with moderate to severe dementia. It causes fewer adverse effects than acetylcholinesterase inhibitors.

► Whether adding memantine to an acetylcholinesterase inhibitor is more effective than an acetylcholinesterase inhibitor alone remains to be established.

► The amyloid beta-directed monoclonal antibody aducanumab can reduce amyloid beta plaques in the brain, but it was not more effective than placebo in slowing cognitive decline in clinical trials.

---

compared to placebo, but few trials have been conducted in patients >85 years old and data on their use for more than one year are limited. Rivastigmine is the only acetylcholinesterase inhibitor FDA-approved for treatment of mild to moderate dementia associated with Parkinson's disease. None of these drugs are approved for treatment of dementia with Lewy bodies or vascular dementia.

Dose-related GI adverse effects (nausea, vomiting, diarrhea) are common with oral acetylcholinesterase inhibitors. Bradycardia and syncope can occur, and an increased incidence of falls and hip fractures has been reported in elderly patients taking these drugs. Because of their cholinergic effects, they should be used with caution in patients who are at an increased risk for peptic ulcer disease and/or GI bleeding and in those with asthma or chronic obstructive pulmonary disease (COPD).

DONEPEZIL — Donepezil (*Aricept*, and others) is a reversible inhibitor of acetylcholinesterase. It is FDA-approved for all stages of AD dementia.

Pharmacokinetics – Oral donepezil is rapidly absorbed from the GI tract; plasma concentrations peak in 3-4 hours with the 10-mg tablet and in about 8 hours with the 23-mg tablet. In healthy subjects, donepezil exposure with the 10 mg/day transdermal formulation was similar to that with 10-mg tablets.[3] The half-life of donepezil is about 70 hours with oral tablets and about 91 hours with transdermal patches. The drug is metabolized primarily by CYP2D6 and 3A4 and is excreted in urine. Higher plasma levels of the drug may occur in CYP2D6 poor metabolizers.

Clinical Studies – In a randomized, double-blind trial comparing oral donepezil 10 mg/day, vitamin E 2000 IU/day, and placebo in 769 patients with **mild cognitive impairment (MCI)**, there were no significant differences between the treatment groups in the probability of progression to AD at 3 years. The donepezil group had a lower rate of progression to AD during the first year of treatment, but after 3 years the rate of progression with donepezil was similar to the rate with placebo. Carriers of the ApoE4 gene had more sustained benefits with donepezil.[4]

In short-term, randomized, double-blind, placebo-controlled trials in patients with **mild to moderate AD**, oral donepezil 5 or 10 mg/day improved cognition and global functioning.[5,6] In a randomized, double-blind, placebo-controlled, 3-year trial, however, in 565 patients with mild to moderate AD, oral donepezil demonstrated no significant benefits on institutionalization or progression of disability.[7]

In a randomized, double-blind, 24-week trial in patients with **moderate to severe AD**, 23 mg/day of oral donepezil improved cognition compared to 10 mg/day, but also had a higher incidence of GI adverse effects.[8]

In a randomized, double-blind, 24-week trial in 248 patients with **severe AD** living in assisted-care facilities, oral donepezil improved activities of daily living, cognition, and global functioning compared to placebo.[9] In a randomized, double-blind, 24-week trial in 343 ambulatory outpatients with severe AD, oral donepezil was more effective than placebo in improving cognition and global functioning.[10]

The results of some small, short-term (10-26 weeks), placebo-controlled trials have suggested a modest improvement in cognition, global functioning,

Table 1. Drugs for Alzheimer's Disease

Drugs	Formulations
Acetylcholinesterase Inhibitors	
Donepezil – generic *Aricept* (Eisai)	5, 10, 23 mg tabs[2]
orally disintegrating – generic	5, 10 mg orally disintegrating tabs
transdermal – *Adlarity* (Corium)	5, 10 mg/24 hr patches
Galantamine – generic	4, 8, 12 mg tabs; 4 mg/mL soln
extended-release – generic *Razadyne ER* (Janssen)	8, 16, 24 mg ER caps
Rivastigmine – generic	1.5, 3, 4.5, 6 mg caps
transdermal – generic *Exelon Patch* (Novartis)	4.6, 9.5, 13.3 mg/24 hr patches
NMDA-Receptor Antagonist	
Memantine – generic *Namenda* (Allergan)	5, 10 mg tabs; 2 mg/mL soln 5, 10 mg tabs
extended-release – generic *Namenda XR*	7, 14, 21, 28 mg ER caps[9]

ER = extended-release
1. Approximate WAC for 28 days' treatment. Cost of aducanumab is for a 70-kg patient. WAC = wholesaler acquisition cost or manufacturer's published price to wholesalers; WAC represents a published catalogue or list price and may not represent an actual transactional price. Source: AnalySource® Monthly. July 5, 2022. Reprinted with permission by First Databank, Inc. All rights reserved. ©2022. www.fdbhealth.com/drug-pricing-policy.
2. The 23-mg tablet should not be split, crushed, or chewed. The 23-mg dose may cause more GI adverse effects.
3. Maximum dose of oral donepezil is 10 mg/day in patients with mild to moderate AD and 23 mg/day in those with moderate to severe disease.

Starting Adult Dosage	Usual Adult Dosage	Cost[1]
5 mg PO once/day; after 4-6 wks increase to 10 mg once/day; after an additional 3 months can increase to 23 mg once/day[3]	5-10 mg PO once/day in the evening	$3.00 506.10 31.90
5 mg/day applied once/wk; after 4-6 wks can increase to 10 mg/day	5 or 10 mg/day applied once/wk[4]	450.00
4 mg PO bid[5]; after 4 wks increase to 8 mg bid; after an additional 4 wks can increase to 12 mg bid	8-12 mg PO bid[5,6]	39.30
8 mg PO once/day[5]; after 4 wks increase to 16 mg once/day; after an additional 4 wks can increase to 24 mg once/day	16-24 mg PO once/day in the morning[5,6]	137.50 320.20
1.5 mg PO bid[5]; increase in increments of 1.5 mg bid every 2 wks[7] to 6 mg bid	4.5-6 mg PO bid[5]	20.00
4.6 mg/day applied q24 hrs; after 4 wks increase to 9.5 mg/day; after an additional 4 wks can increase to 13.3 mg/day	9.5 or 13.3 mg/day applied q24 hrs	305.80 686.00
5 mg PO once/day; increase in increments of 5 mg/wk to 10 mg bid	10 mg PO bid[8]	13.00 444.80
7 mg PO once/day; increase in increments of 7 mg/wk to 28 mg once/day	28 mg PO once/day[8]	136.90 464.80

4. Maximum dose of transdermal donepezil is 10 mg/day.
5. Taken with meals.
6. In patients with CrCl 9-59 mL/min or moderate hepatic impairment, dosage should not exceed 16 mg/day. Patients with CrCl <9 mL/min or severe hepatic impairment should not take galantamine.
7. Every 4 weeks for dementia associated with Parkinson's disease.
8. In patients with severe renal impairment (CrCl 5-29 mL/min), the target dosage is 5 mg bid for the immediate-release formulation and 14 mg once/day for the extended-release formulation.
9. Contents of capsules can be sprinkled on applesauce and consumed immediately. Capsules should not be divided, crushed, or chewed.

Continued on next page

Table 1. Drugs for Alzheimer's Disease (continued)	
Drugs	**Formulations**
NMDA-Receptor Antagonist/Acetylcholinesterase Inhibitor	
Memantine/donepezil – Namzaric (Allergan)[10]	7/10, 14/10, 21/10, 28/10 mg ER caps[9]
Amyloid Beta-Directed Monoclonal Antibody	
Aducanumab – Aduhelm (Biogen/Eisai)	170 mg/1.7 mL, 300 mg/3 mL single dose vials

ER = extended-release
10. Approved for patients previously stabilized on donepezil 10 mg once/day.
11. For patients who were taking donepezil 10 mg once/day without memantine, the recommended starting dosage is 7/10 mg once/day in the evening; the memantine daily dose can be increased in increments of 7 mg/week. For patients previously stabilized on donepezil 10 mg once/day and memantine 10 mg bid or 28 mg once/day, the recommended starting dosage is 28/10 mg once/day in the evening.

and activities of daily living with oral donepezil in patients with **dementia associated with Parkinson's disease** or **dementia with Lewy bodies**.[11] In one placebo-controlled trial, donepezil improved cognition and global functioning in patients with **vascular dementia**.[12]

FDA approval of the transdermal formulation of donepezil *(Adlarity)* for treatment of all stages of AD dementia was based on the results of previous studies with oral donepezil tablets and a pharmacokinetic study showing that the bioavailability of the transdermal formulation is similar to that of the oral formulation.[13] No trials comparing the efficacy and tolerability of transdermal and oral donepezil are available.

Adverse Effects – The most common adverse effects of oral donepezil are nausea, vomiting, diarrhea, anorexia, fatigue, and muscle cramps; these effects generally resolve with continued treatment. In healthy subjects treated with transdermal donepezil, the most common adverse effects were headache, application-site pruritus, dermatitis and pain,

Starting Adult Dosage	Usual Adult Dosage	Cost[1]
See footnote 11	28/10 mg PO once/day in the evening[12]	$535.60
1 mg/kg IV q4 wks for infusions 1 and 2, 3 mg/kg q4 wks for infusions 3 and 4, 6 mg/kg q4 wks for infusions 5 and 6, and 10 mg/kg q4 wks for infusion 7 and beyond	10 mg/kg IV q4 wks	2171.40

12. The recommended dosage of *Namzaric* is 14/10 mg once/day for patients with severe renal impairment (CrCl 5-29 mL/min) previously stabilized on memantine 5 mg bid or 14 mg once/day and donepezil 10 mg once/day.

muscle spasms, insomnia, abdominal pain, constipation, diarrhea, dizziness, abnormal dreams, and skin laceration.

Drug Interactions – Use of donepezil with other drugs that have cholinergic effects can result in additive toxicity. Drugs that have anticholinergic properties can antagonize the effects of donepezil. Donepezil may interact with inhibitors of CYP3A4 or 2D6 or with inducers of CYP3A4.[14]

GALANTAMINE — Galantamine (*Razadyne ER*, and generics) is a reversible competitive inhibitor of acetylcholinesterase. It also acts on nicotinic acetylcholine receptors, but the clinical significance of its nicotinic activity remains to be established. Galantamine is FDA-approved for treatment of mild to moderate AD dementia.

Pharmacokinetics – Galantamine is rapidly absorbed from the GI tract. Serum concentrations of the immediate-release formulation peak in about 1 hour when taken without food and in about 2.5 hours when taken with food. Serum concentrations of the extended-release formulation peak in 4.5-5 hours. Galantamine has a half-life of about 7 hours. It is metabolized by CYP2D6 to an active metabolite that is more potent than the parent drug in inhibiting acetylcholinesterase and by CYP3A4 to metabolites that have little anticholinesterase activity. Higher plasma levels of galantamine may occur in CYP2D6 poor metabolizers.

Clinical Studies – In two randomized, 2-year trials in a total of 2048 patients with **MCI**, there was no significant difference in the rate of progression to AD between galantamine- and placebo-treated patients.[15]

In short-term (4-6 months) trials in patients with **mild to moderate AD**, galantamine modestly improved cognitive and global functioning compared to placebo.[16-18] In a randomized, placebo-controlled, 2-year trial in 2045 patients with mild to moderate AD, the mortality rate was lower in galantamine-treated patients and cognitive and functional impairment were worse in placebo-treated patients.[19] In a post-hoc analysis, patients taking memantine did not benefit from addition of galantamine.[20]

Two trials (6-12 months) in patients with AD and/or **cerebrovascular disease** showed improvements in cognition, global functioning, behavior, and activities of daily living with galantamine treatment.[21,22]

Adverse Effects – Nausea, vomiting, diarrhea, dizziness, headache, and weight loss are common with rapid dose escalation of galantamine, but are less common during maintenance treatment. Depression, fatigue, and somnolence have been reported.

Drug Interactions – Use of galantamine with other drugs that have cholinergic effects can result in additive toxicity. Drugs that have anticholinergic properties can antagonize the effects of galantamine. Galantamine may interact with drugs that inhibit CYP3A4 or 2D6 or induce CYP3A4.[14]

RIVASTIGMINE — Rivastigmine is a carbamate-based, slowly reversible, noncompetitive acetylcholinesterase inhibitor. It is FDA-approved for treatment of mild to moderate dementia associated with AD or Parkinson's disease. The transdermal patch formulation (*Exelon Patch*, and generics) is also FDA-approved for severe AD dementia.

Pharmacokinetics – The oral formulation of rivastigmine is rapidly absorbed from the GI tract; plasma concentrations peak in about 1 hour when taken without food and in about 2.5 hours when taken with food. The drug binds weakly to plasma proteins and has a short half-life in plasma (1.5 hours), but its half-life for cholinesterase inhibition in the CNS is about 10 hours. Rivastigmine is primarily metabolized through hydrolysis by esterases and is excreted in urine.

Clinical Studies – In a randomized, double-blind trial of up to 48 months duration in 1018 patients with **MCI**, there was no significant difference in cognitive function or rate of progression to AD between rivastigmine and placebo.[23]

A review of 13 randomized, double-blind, placebo-controlled, 12- to 52-week trials in 4775 patients with **mild to moderate AD** found that oral and transdermal rivastigmine slowed the rate of cognitive decline and improved activities of daily living, but the effects were modest and the clinical significance was unclear. The transdermal patch was associated with a lower rate of GI adverse effects than the oral formulation.[24]

In a 24-week trial in 1195 patients with **probable AD**, transdermal rivastigmine (9.5 mg/24 hours) was similar in efficacy to oral rivastigmine (12 mg/day), and the incidence of nausea and vomiting was about two-thirds lower with the patch.[25] In a 24-week trial, 716 patients with **severe AD** were randomized to receive either 4.6 or 13.3 mg/24 hours of transdermal rivastigmine; mean declines from baseline on assessments of cognition and overall function were statistically significantly less with the 13.3-mg patch.[26]

In a randomized, double-blind, placebo-controlled, 24-week trial in 28 patients with **dementia associated with Parkinson's disease**, transdermal rivastigmine produced improvements in attention and cognition.[27] In a randomized, double-blind, placebo-controlled, 20-week trial in 120 patients with **dementia with Lewy bodies**, oral rivastigmine produced improvements in behavior.[28] In a randomized, double-blind, 24-week trial in 710 patients with probable **vascular dementia**, oral rivastigmine improved measures of cognition, but not global impression of change or activities of daily living.[29]

Adverse Effects – Oral rivastigmine commonly causes nausea, vomiting, and diarrhea; GI tolerability can be improved with slow titration and by taking the drug with food. These effects appear to occur less frequently with the transdermal formulation.

Drug Interactions – Use of rivastigmine with other drugs that have cholinergic effects can result in additive toxicity. Drugs that have anticholinergic properties can antagonize the effects of rivastigmine.

CHOICE OF A CHOLINESTERASE INHIBITOR — Most studies of cholinesterase inhibitors demonstrate modest improvements in cognitive and functional measures, but improvements in behavior are less consistent. Donepezil, galantamine, and rivastigmine appear to be similar in efficacy and safety in patients with AD, but randomized controlled trials comparing these drugs are lacking. A matched cohort study of patients from the Swedish Dementia Registry found that use of any of the cholinesterase inhibitors was associated with a reduction in cognitive decline and a lower risk of death; galantamine use was associated with lower rates of cognitive decline and mortality than donepezil and rivastigmine.[30] Transdermal formulations of donepezil and rivastigmine may be better tolerated than the oral formulations. Both donepezil and rivastigmine have documented efficacy in dementia associated with Parkinson's disease and dementia with Lewy bodies. Donepezil, rivastigmine, and galantamine have improved cognitive performance in patients with vascular dementia.

AN NMDA-RECEPTOR ANTAGONIST

MEMANTINE — An N-methyl-D-aspartate (NMDA) receptor antagonist, memantine (*Namenda*, and others) is FDA-approved for treatment of moderate to severe AD dementia. Its mechanism of action in AD is unclear; it may reduce glutamatergic overstimulation at the NMDA receptor, which could have symptomatic benefits.[31] Memantine is available in an extended-release, fixed-dose combination with donepezil *(Namzaric)* that is FDA-approved for once-daily treatment of moderate to severe AD dementia.

Pharmacokinetics – Memantine is well absorbed from the GI tract. Plasma concentrations peak in about 3-7 hours with the immediate-release formulation and about 9-12 hours with the extended-release formulation. The terminal elimination half-life is 60-80 hours. Memantine is excreted primarily in urine.

Clinical Studies – A recent meta-analysis of 15 trials in about 3700 patients with **moderate to severe AD** found a small but consistent benefit for memantine versus placebo in cognitive function, activities of daily living, behavior, and mood.[32]

In a prospective, double-blind, 24-week trial in 433 patients with **mild to moderate AD** taking an acetylcholinesterase inhibitor, addition of memantine was no more effective than addition of placebo.[33]

In one randomized trial in 404 patients with **moderate to severe AD** taking donepezil, addition of memantine led to better outcomes on measures of cognition, behavior, activities of daily living, and global outcomes compared to addition of placebo.[34] In another randomized trial, however, in 295 patients with moderate to severe AD taking donepezil, addition of memantine did not significantly improve measures of cognition and activities of daily living compared to addition of placebo.[35]

There is no acceptable evidence that memantine is effective in **mild AD**.

Memantine has been reported to improve cognition in patients with mild to moderate **vascular dementia**.[36,37] It has not been shown to be effective in **Parkinson's disease dementia** or **dementia with Lewy bodies**.[38]

Adverse Effects – Memantine is usually well tolerated. Confusion, agitation, dizziness, insomnia, hallucinations, and delusions can occur.

Drug Interactions – Memantine does not affect the activity of acetylcholinesterase inhibitors. Amantadine, which is used to treat Parkinson's disease, is also an NMDA-receptor antagonist; taking it with memantine could theoretically result in undesirable additive effects.

AN AMYLOID BETA-DIRECTED MONOCLONAL ANTIBODY

Aducanumab *(Aduhelm)*, an IV amyloid beta-directed monoclonal antibody, is FDA-approved for treatment of MCI or mild dementia due to AD.[39,40] The approval was based on the surrogate endpoint of reduction in amyloid beta plaques in the brain, but the role of amyloid beta plaques in the pathogenesis of cognitive decline is unclear; multiple large clinical trials with other agents have failed to demonstrate that reducing amyloid beta plaques in the brains of patients with AD results in a meaningful clinical benefit. The Centers for Medicare and Medicaid Services (CMS) has announced that it will pay for aducanumab for treatment of AD only in patients enrolled in a qualifying clinical trial.[41]

Clinical Studies – In two double-blind trials in a total of 3285 patients with **early AD**, patients were randomized to receive low- or high-dose aducanumab or placebo IV every 4 weeks for 18 months. Both trials were terminated early after an initial analysis concluded that the drug was not more effective than placebo in slowing cognitive decline. In one trial, but not the other, a post-hoc analysis found that the highest dose of aducanumab was associated with statistically significant improvements from baseline in tests of cognitive and functional outcomes compared to placebo.[42,43]

PET imaging was used to evaluate the effect of aducanumab on brain amyloid beta plaque in a total of 1073 patients from the two clinical trials and in a separate 54-week dose-ranging trial in 197 patients with mild dementia. In all three studies, treatment with aducanumab significantly reduced amyloid beta plaque compared to placebo.

Adverse Effects – Serial MRIs detected cerebral edema in 35%, micro-hemorrhages in 19%, and superficial siderosis in 15% of patients treated with high-dose aducanumab in the two clinical trials. Titrating the dose decreases the incidence and severity of these amyloid-related imaging abnormalities (ARIA), the principal adverse effects of the drug; regular MRI safety scans should be performed. These abnormalities can be accompanied by headache, dizziness, unsteadiness, confusion, visual changes and, rarely, seizures. One fatality related to ARIA has been reported. Carriers of the ApoE4 gene have a higher incidence of ARIA.[44]

ANTIPSYCHOTICS

Antipsychotic drugs are widely used off-label to treat agitation and other behavioral symptoms in elderly patients, especially those with dementia. Second-generation antipsychotic drugs used in low doses have generally been preferred over first-generation drugs because they are less likely to cause extrapyramidal effects.[45]

Efficacy in AD Dementia – Although many clinicians believe that use of second-generation antipsychotics such as quetiapine (*Seroquel*, and generics) to calm agitated or aggressive patients with dementia is beneficial, evidence from randomized controlled trials is limited. In one randomized, placebo-controlled, 36-week trial in 421 outpatients with AD, treatment with an antipsychotic modestly improved behavioral symptoms such as anger, aggression, and paranoid ideation, but did not improve functioning, care needs, or quality of life.[46]

Pimavanserin – A second-generation antipsychotic drug with no structural resemblance to other antipsychotic drugs and no clinically significant effects on dopaminergic, adrenergic, histaminic, or muscarinic receptors, pimavanserin (*Nuplazid*, and generics) is FDA-approved for treatment of hallucinations and delusions associated with Parkinson's disease.[47] It is an inverse agonist and antagonist at serotonin 5-HT$_{2A}$ receptors, which have been implicated in the development of hallucinations and delusions in patients with Parkinson's disease. A discontinuation trial in patients with any dementia-related psychosis found that those who responded to pimavanserin in an open-label trial (62%) had a lower risk of relapse with continuation of the drug than with substitution of placebo.[48]

Adverse Effects – Common adverse effects of antipsychotic drugs include somnolence and gait changes. Extrapyramidal effects can occur and may be more severe in patients also taking an acetylcholinesterase inhibitor.[49] In one study in 421 patients with AD, cognitive function declined more in patients taking an antipsychotic drug than in those taking placebo.[50] Pimavanserin does not cause somnolence, gait changes, or extrapyramidal effects, but it does prolong the QT interval and should not be used in patients with hepatic or severe renal impairment.

Risk of Death – The FDA requires manufacturers of all antipsychotic drugs to include a warning in the labeling about an increased risk of death among elderly patients with dementia treated with antipsychotic drugs. In randomized trials, elderly patients with dementia taking second-generation antipsychotic drugs had a higher mortality rate than those taking placebo (4.5% vs 2.6% in a typical 10-week controlled trial); most of the deaths were attributed to cardiovascular or infectious causes. The mortality risk with first-generation antipsychotic drugs has not been adequately evaluated and may be higher than the risk with second-generation drugs.

ANTIDEPRESSANTS

Antidepressant drugs are used off-label to treat agitation and other behavioral symptoms in patients with dementia. A review of 9 trials in a total of 692 patients with dementia found that the selective serotonin reuptake inhibitors (SSRIs) sertraline (*Zoloft*, and generics) and citalopram (*Celexa*, and generics) improved agitation, but not other behavioral symptoms.[51] In a randomized, double-blind, 9-week trial in 186 patients with AD and clinically significant agitation, citalopram improved measures of agitation compared to placebo, but it was also associated with worsening of cognition and QT-interval prolongation.[52]

OTHER DRUGS

Dextromethorphan/quinidine *(Nuedexta)* is FDA-approved for treatment of pseudobulbar affect, which occurs in a range of neurological disorders.[53] Quinidine is a strong CYP2D6 inhibitor[14]; it increases serum concentrations of the CYP2D6 substrate dextromethorphan. In a randomized, placebo-controlled trial in 194 patients with AD-related agitation, measures of agitation and aggression were modestly improved in those receiving the combination. Adverse effects were infrequent, but included dizziness, falls, diarrhea, and urinary tract infection.[54]

A randomized trial in 613 patients with mild to moderate AD compared 2000 IU/day of **vitamin E**, 20 mg of memantine, a combination of both vitamin E and memantine, and placebo. Compared to placebo, functional decline was statistically significantly slower with vitamin E, but not with memantine or the combination of vitamin E and memantine.[55] A long-term prevention study of antioxidant supplements found that vitamin E did not prevent dementia.[56]

The dietary supplement **Ginkgo biloba** is heavily promoted in the US for memory support. In several randomized, double-blind trials, it was not effective in preventing or treating dementia or for preventing cognitive decline in older adults.[57-59]

The dietary supplement *Prevagen*, which contains a synthetic form of the protein **apoaequorin**, is heavily marketed to improve memory. There is no acceptable evidence that the drug is effective for memory improvement; patients should be advised not to take it.[60]

1. DS Knopman et al. Alzheimer disease. Nat Rev Dis Primers 2021; 7:33.
2. G Marucci et al. Efficacy of acetylcholinesterase inhibitors in Alzheimer's disease. Neuropharmacology 2021; 190:108352.
3. A donepezil patch (Adlarity) for Alzheimer's disease. Med Lett Drugs Ther 2022; 64:e128.
4. RC Petersen et al. Vitamin E and donepezil for the treatment of mild cognitive impairment. N Engl J Med 2005; 352:2379.

5. SL Rogers et al. A 24-week, double-blind, placebo-controlled trial of donepezil in patients with Alzheimer's disease. Neurology 1998; 50:136.
6. SL Rogers and LT Friedhoff. The efficacy and safety of donepezil in patients with Alzheimer's disease: results of a US multicentre, randomized, double-blind, placebo-controlled trial. Dementia 1996; 7:293.
7. C Courtney et al. Long-term donepezil treatment in 565 patients with Alzheimer's disease (AD2000): randomised double-blind trial. Lancet 2004; 363:2105.
8. MR Farlow et al. Effectiveness and tolerability of high-dose (23 mg/day) versus standard-dose (10 mg/day) donepezil in moderate to severe Alzheimer's disease: a 24-week, randomized, double-blind study. Clin Ther 2010; 32:1234.
9. B Winblad et al. Donepezil in patients with severe Alzheimer's disease: double-blind, parallel-group, placebo-controlled study. Lancet 2006; 367:1057.
10. SE Black et al. Donepezil preserves cognition and global function in patients with severe Alzheimer disease. Neurology 2007; 69:459.
11. M Rolinski et al. Cholinesterase inhibitors for dementia with Lewy bodies, Parkinson's disease dementia and cognitive impairment in Parkinson's disease. Cochrane Database Syst Rev 2012; 3:CD006504.
12. D Wilkinson et al. Donepezil in vascular dementia: a randomized, placebo-controlled study. Neurology 2003; 61:479.
13. SK Yoon et al. Pharmacokinetic evaluation by modeling and simulation analysis of a donepezil patch formulation in healthy male volunteers. Drug Des Devel Ther 2020; 14:1729.
14. Inhibitors and inducers of CYP enzymes, P-glycoprotein, and other transporters. Med Lett Drugs Ther 2021 October 20 (epub). Available at: medicalletter.org/downloads/ CYP_PGP_Tables.pdf.
15. B Winblad et al. Safety and efficacy of galantamine in subjects with mild cognitive impairment. Neurology 2008; 70:2024.
16. K Rockwood et al. Attainment of treatment goals by people with Alzheimer's disease receiving galantamine: a randomized controlled trial. CMAJ 2006; 174:1099.
17. GK Wilcock et al. Efficacy and safety of galantamine in patients with mild to moderate Alzheimer's disease: multicentre randomised controlled trial. BMJ 2000; 321:1445.
18. PN Tariot et al. A 5-month, randomized, placebo-controlled trial of galantamine in AD. Neurology 2000; 54:2269.
19. K Hager et al. Effects of galantamine in a 2-year, randomized, placebo-controlled study in Alzheimer's disease. Neuropsychiatr Dis Treat 2014; 10:391.
20. K Hager et al. Effect of concomitant use of memantine on mortality and efficacy outcomes of galantamine-treated patients with Alzheimer's disease: post-hoc analysis of a randomized placebo-controlled study. Alzheimers Res Ther 2016; 8:47.
21. T Erkinjuntti et al. Efficacy of galantamine in probable vascular dementia and Alzheimer's disease combined with cerebrovascular disease: a randomised trial. Lancet 2002; 359:1283.
22. R Bullock et al. Management of patients with Alzheimer's disease plus cerebrovascular disease: 12-month treatment with galantamine. Dement Geriatr Cogn Disord 2004; 17:29.
23. HH Feldman et al. Effect of rivastigmine on delay to diagnosis of Alzheimer's disease from mild cognitive impairment: the InDDEx study. Lancet Neurol 2007; 6:501.

24. JS Birks et al. Rivastigmine for Alzheimer's disease. Cochrane Database Syst Rev 2015; 9:CD001191.
25. B Winblad et al. A six-month double-blind, randomized, placebo-controlled study of a transdermal patch in Alzheimer's disease – rivastigmine patch versus capsule. Int J Geriatr Psychiatry 2007; 22:456.
26. MR Fárlow et al. A 24-week, randomized, controlled trial of rivastigmine patch 13.3 mg/24 h versus 4.6 mg/24 h in severe Alzheimer's dementia. CNS Neurosci Ther 2013; 19:745.
27. E Mamikonyan et al. Rivastigmine for mild cognitive impairment in Parkinson disease: a placebo-controlled study. Mov Disord 2015; 30:912.
28. I McKeith et al. Efficacy of rivastigmine in dementia with Lewy bodies: a randomised, double-blind, placebo-controlled international study. Lancet 2000; 356:2031.
29. C Ballard et al. Efficacy, safety and tolerability of rivastigmine capsules in patients with probable vascular dementia: the VantagE study. Curr Med Res Opin 2008; 24:2561.
30. H Xu et al. Long-term effects of cholinesterase inhibitors on cognitive decline and mortality. Neurology 2021; 96:e2220.
31. PT Francis et al. Rationale for combining glutamatergic and cholinergic approaches in the symptomatic treatment of Alzheimer's disease. Expert Rev Neurother 2012; 12:1351.
32. R McShane et al. Memantine for dementia. Cochrane Database Syst Rev 2019; 3:CD003154.
33. AP Porsteinsson et al. Memantine treatment in patients with mild to moderate Alzheimer's disease already receiving a cholinesterase inhibitor: a randomized, double-blind, placebo-controlled trial. Curr Alzheimer Res 2008; 5:83.
34. PN Tariot et al. Memantine treatment in patients with moderate to severe Alzheimer disease already receiving donepezil: a randomized controlled trial. JAMA 2004; 291:317.
35. R Howard et al. Donepezil and memantine for moderate-to-severe Alzheimer's disease. N Engl J Med 2012; 366:893.
36. JM Orgogozo et al. Efficacy and safety of memantine in patients with mild to moderate vascular dementia: a randomized, placebo-controlled trial (MMM 300). Stroke 2002; 33:1834.
37. G Wilcock et al. A double-blind, placebo-controlled multicentre study of memantine in mild to moderate vascular dementia (MMM500). Int Clin Psychopharmacol 2002; 17:297.
38. HF Wang et al. Efficacy and safety of cholinesterase inhibitors and memantine in cognitive impairment in Parkinson's disease, Parkinson's disease dementia, and dementia with Lewy bodies: systematic review with meta-analysis and trial sequential analysis. J Neurol Neurosurg Psychiatry 2015; 86:135.
39. Aducanumab (Aduhelm) for Alzheimer's disease. Med Lett Drugs Ther 2021; 63:105.
40. GC Alexander et al. Revisiting FDA approval of aducanumab. N Engl J Med 2021; 385:769.
41. J Stephenson. Medicare to cover controversial Alzheimer disease drug only in clinical trials. JAMA Health Forum 2022; 3:e220048.
42. S Salloway et al. Amyloid-related imaging abnormalities in 2 phase 3 studies evaluating aducanumab in patients with early Alzheimer disease. JAMA Neurol 2022; 79:13.
43. SB Haeberlein et al. Two randomized phase 3 studies of aducanumab in early Alzheimer's disease. J Prev Alzheimers Dis 2022; 9:197.

44. J Cummings et al. Aducanumab: appropriate use recommendations. J Prev Alzheimers Dis 2021; 8:398.

45. VI Reus et al. The American Psychiatric Association practice guideline on the use of antipsychotics to treat agitation or psychosis in patients with dementia. Am J Psychiatry 2016; 173:543.

46. DL Sultzer et al. Clinical symptom responses to atypical antipsychotic medications in Alzheimer's disease: phase 1 outcomes from the CATIE-AD effectiveness trial. Am J Psychiatry 2008; 165:844.

47. Drugs for Parkinson's disease. Med Lett Drugs Ther 2021; 63:25.

48. PN Tariot et al. Trial of pimavanserin in dementia-related psychosis. N Engl J Med 2021; 385:309.

49. HC Liu et al. Extrapyramidal side-effect due to drug combination of risperidone and donepezil. Psychiatry Clin Neurosci 2002; 56:479.

50. CLP Vigen et al. Cognitive effects of atypical antipsychotic medications in patients with Alzheimer's disease: outcomes from CATIE-AD. Am J Psychiatry 2011; 168:831.

51. DP Seitz et al. Antidepressants for agitation and psychosis in dementia. Cochrane Database Syst Rev 2011; 2:CD008191.

52. AP Porsteinsson et al. Effect of citalopram on agitation in Alzheimer disease: the CitAD randomized clinical trial. JAMA 2014; 311:682.

53. Dextromethorphan/quinidine (Nuedexta) for pseudobulbar affect. Med Lett Drugs Ther 2011; 53:46.

54. JL Cummings et al. Effect of dextromethorphan-quinidine on agitation in patients with Alzheimer disease dementia: a randomized clinical trial. JAMA 2015; 314:1242.

55. MW Dysken et al. Effect of vitamin E and memantine on functional decline in Alzheimer disease: the TEAM-AD VA cooperative randomized trial. JAMA 2014; 311:33.

56. RJ Kryscio et al. Association of antioxidant supplement use and dementia in the prevention of Alzheimer's disease by vitamin E and selenium trial (PREADViSE). JAMA Neurol 2017; 74:567.

57. LS Schneider et al. A randomized, double-blind, placebo-controlled trial of two doses of Ginkgo biloba extract in dementia of the Alzheimer's type. Curr Alzheimer Res 2005; 2:541.

58. BE Snitz et al. Ginkgo biloba for preventing cognitive decline in older adults: a randomized trial. JAMA 2009; 302:2663.

59. B Vellas et al. Long-term use of standardized Ginkgo biloba extract for the prevention of Alzheimer's disease (GuidAge): a randomised placebo-controlled trial. Lancet Neurol 2012; 11:851.

60. Apoaequorin (Prevagen) to improve memory. Med Lett Drugs Ther 2021; 63:175.

DRUGS FOR
Type 2 Diabetes

Original publication date – November 2022

Diet, exercise, and weight loss can improve glycemic control, but almost all patients with type 2 diabetes require antihyperglycemic drug therapy. Treating to a target A1C of <7% while minimizing hypoglycemia is recommended to prevent microvascular complications of diabetes (retinopathy, nephropathy, and neuropathy). An A1C target of <8% may be appropriate for some older patients.[1]

Metformin is generally preferred for initial treatment of type 2 diabetes, but an SGLT2 inhibitor or a GLP-1 receptor agonist may be added or substituted in some patients.[1] Many patients require insulin for glycemic control; insulin therapy for type 2 diabetes was reviewed in a previous issue.[2]

METFORMIN — The oral biguanide metformin is generally preferred for initial treatment of type 2 diabetes. Metformin decreases hepatic glucose production and increases secretion of GLP-1. It may also reduce intestinal absorption of glucose and (to a lesser extent) increase peripheral glucose uptake. Metformin monotherapy reduces A1C by 1-1.5%, is weight-neutral or causes modest weight loss, and does not cause hypoglycemia.

The FDA has moderated its warning against use of metformin in patients with renal impairment. Metformin is still contraindicated for use in patients with an eGFR <30 mL/min/1.73 m^2, and starting the drug in patients with an eGFR of 30-45 mL/min/1.73 m^2 is not recommended.[3] In a series of

Abbreviation Key
ASCVD = atherosclerotic cardiovascular disease
CKD = chronic kidney disease
CV = cardiovascular
CVD = cardiovascular disease
DPP-4 = dipeptidyl peptidase-4
GIP = glucose-dependent insulinotropic polypeptide
GLP-1 = glucagon-like peptide-1
HF = heart failure
MACE = major adverse cardiovascular events
SGLT2 = sodium-glucose cotransporter 2

retrospective cohort studies in a total of ~49,000 patients with type 2 diabetes who continued taking metformin or a sulfonylurea after developing renal impairment, rates of MACE and hospitalization for HF were lower with metformin than with sulfonylurea monotherapy and rates of lactic acidosis were similar with both drugs.[4-6]

Adding a Second Drug – The choice of a second antihyperglycemic drug is generally based on the presence of comorbid conditions such as ASCVD, HF, CKD, and obesity. In a meta-analysis of 8 cardiovascular outcomes trials in patients with type 2 diabetes, SGLT2 inhibitors and GLP-1 receptor agonists reduced MACE to a similar extent (11-12%) in patients with established ASCVD. SGLT2 inhibitors were more effective than GLP-1 receptor agonists in preventing hospitalization for HF and progression of kidney disease.[7]

In most patients without CVD, HF, or CKD, lowering A1C while minimizing hypoglycemia is the main goal of treatment. The recently published GRADE trial evaluated the comparative effectiveness of 4 antihyperglycemic drugs (insulin glargine, the sulfonylurea glimepiride, the GLP-1 receptor agonist liraglutide, and the DDP-4 inhibitor sitagliptin) added to metformin in reducing A1C. An SGLT2 inhibitor was not included because none had been approved by the FDA at the time the trial began. Over a mean follow-up of 5 years, patients in the insulin glargine and

---

Key Points: Drugs for Type 2 Diabetes

▸ Treating to a target A1C of <7% while minimizing hypoglycemia is recommended to prevent microvascular complications of type 2 diabetes (<8% may be appropriate for some patients).

▸ Most patients require multidrug regimens to achieve their A1C goal.

▸ Metformin is generally preferred for initial treatment.

▸ Patients with atherosclerotic cardiovascular disease, heart failure, or chronic kidney disease may benefit from addition of an SGLT2 inhibitor or a GLP-1 receptor agonist with proven cardiovascular or renal benefits.

▸ GLP-1 receptor agonists, SGLT2 inhibitors, and tirzepatide are beneficial for patients who require weight loss.

---

liraglutide groups were statistically significantly more likely to achieve and maintain an A1C of ≤7.0%.[8] The rates of MACE, hospitalization for HF, CV death, albuminuria, and neuropathy were about the same in all 4 groups.[9]

In other trials, addition of the oral GLP-1 receptor agonist semaglutide to standard treatment was superior to addition of the SGLT2 inhibitor empagliflozin or the DPP-4 inhibitor sitagliptin and noninferior to addition of liraglutide in reducing A1C.[10-13]

SGLT2 INHIBITORS — Sodium-glucose cotransporter 2 inhibitors decrease renal glucose reabsorption and increase urinary glucose excretion, reducing fasting and postprandial blood glucose levels. Added to standard treatment, canagliflozin, dapagliflozin, and empagliflozin have reduced the risk of MACE and hospitalization for HF and slowed progression of CKD.[14-20] In one double-blind trial in patients with type 2 diabetes and ASCVD, ertugliflozin did not reduce the risk of MACE.[21]

GLP-1 RECEPTOR AGONISTS — Glucagon-like peptide-1 receptor agonists potentiate glucose-dependent secretion of insulin, suppress glucagon secretion, slow gastric emptying, and promote satiety. Dulaglutide, liraglutide, and subcutaneously injected semaglutide have been shown to reduce the risk of MACE in adults with established CVD

Table 1. Preferred Antihyperglycemic Drugs	
Patient	Preferred Drug[1]
ASCVD/high risk of ASCVD	GLP-1 receptor agonist[2] or SGLT2 inhibitor[3]
HF	SGLT2 inhibitor
CKD	SGLT2 inhibitor[4]
Overweight/obese	GLP-1 receptor agonist, SGLT2 inhibitor, or tirzepatide
Needs substantial A1C lowering	Insulin, GLP-1 receptor agonist, sulfonylurea, or tirzepatide
Needs to minimize hypoglycemia	DPP-4 inhibitor, GLP-1 receptor agonist, SGLT2 inhibitor, or thiazolidinedione
Cost/access concerns	Insulin, sulfonylurea, or thiazolidinedione

ASCVD = atherosclerotic cardiovascular disease; CKD = chronic kidney disease; HF = heart failure
1. First-line treatment generally includes metformin.
2. Dulaglutide, liraglutide, or SC semaglutide.
3. Canagliflozin or empagliflozin; data are less robust with dapagliflozin.
4. Canagliflozin, dapagliflozin, or empagliflozin.

and reduce macroalbuminuria, but they have not been shown to reduce hospitalization for HF or slow progression of CKD.[22-27]

Addition of exenatide or lixisenatide to standard treatment has produced mixed results.[28] In one trial in patients with type 2 diabetes with or without CVD, exenatide was not superior to placebo in reducing the incidence of MACE or hospitalization for HF.[29] In patients with type 2 diabetes who had a recent acute coronary event, addition of lixisenatide to standard treatment was not superior to addition of placebo in reducing the rate of MACE or hospitalization for HF.[30]

Subcutaneous semaglutide *(Wegovy)* and liraglutide *(Saxenda)* are FDA-approved for chronic weight management in patients with or without type 2 diabetes in doses higher than those used for treatment of type 2 diabetes.

DUAL GIP/GLP-1 RECEPTOR AGONIST — Tirzepatide is a peptide hormone with activity at both glucose-dependent insulinotropic polypeptide (GIP) and glucagon-like peptide-1 (GLP-1) receptors. In clinical trials in patients with type 2 diabetes, tirzepatide reduced A1C (2-2.5%)

Table 2. FDA-Approved CV and Renal Indications for SGLT2 Inhibitors and GLP-1 Receptor Agonists
SGLT2 Inhibitors
Canagliflozin (Invokana)
▸ Reduce risk of MACE in adults with type 2 diabetes and established CVD
▸ Reduce risk of end-stage kidney disease, doubling of serum creatinine, CV death, and hospitalization for HF in adults with type 2 diabetes and diabetic nephropathy with albuminuria
Dapagliflozin (Farxiga)
▸ Reduce risk of hospitalization for HF in adults with type 2 diabetes and established CVD or multiple CV risk factors
▸ Reduce risk of CV death and hospitalization for HF in adults with HFrEF
▸ Reduce risk of sustained eGFR decline, end-stage kidney disease, CV death, and hospitalization for HF in adults with CKD at risk of progression
Empagliflozin (Jardiance)
▸ Reduce risk of hospitalization for HF and CV death in adults with HF
▸ Reduce risk of CV death in adults with type 2 diabetes and established CVD
GLP-1 Receptor Agonists
Dulaglutide (Trulicity)
▸ Reduce risk of MACE in adults with type 2 diabetes who have established CVD or multiple CV risk factors
Liraglutide (Victoza)
▸ Reduce risk of MACE in adults with type 2 diabetes and established CVD
Semaglutide (Ozempic, Rybelsus)
▸ Reduce risk of MACE in adults with type 2 diabetes and established CVD (only *Ozempic*)
CKD = chronic kidney disease; CV = cardiovascular; CVD = cardiovascular disease; HF = heart failure; HFrEF = heart failure with reduced ejection fraction; MACE = major adverse cardiovascular events

and body weight (7-13 kg) more than placebo, the injectable GLP-1 receptor agonist semaglutide, insulin degludec, and insulin glargine. Cardiovascular outcomes trials with tirzepatide in patients with type 2 diabetes are ongoing.

In a clinical trial in patients without type 2 diabetes, tirzepatide use was associated with significant reductions in weight (15-21%)[31]; it has not yet been approved by the FDA for weight management.

Table 3. Drugs for Type 2 Diabetes

Biguanide (metformin)

A1C reduction: 1.0-1.5%
Hypoglycemia: no, except when also receiving insulin or a sulfonylurea
Weight change: neutral or modest weight loss
CV outcomes: reduced risk of MI and all-cause mortality
Renal: contraindicated with eGFR <30 mL/min/1.73 m^2
Adverse effects: GI (metallic taste, nausea, diarrhea, abdominal pain), possible vitamin B12 deficiency, rarely lactic acidosis

SGLT2 Inhibitors (canagliflozin, dapagliflozin, empagliflozin, ertugliflozin)

A1C reduction: 0.5-1.0%
Hypoglycemia: no, except when also receiving insulin or a sulfonylurea
Weight change: modest weight loss (2-8 kg)
CV outcomes: reduced risk of MACE (empagliflozin, canagliflozin, dapagliflozin); reduced risk of hospitalization for HF (canagliflozin, dapagliflozin, empagliflozin, ertugliflozin)
Renal outcomes: slowed progression of CKD (canagliflozin, dapagliflozin, empagliflozin)
Renal: dosage adjustment required
Adverse effects: genital mycotic infections, urinary tract infections, volume depletion, acute kidney injury, diabetic ketoacidosis, hypotension, possible risk of lower limb amputation (canagliflozin, ertugliflozin), risk of bone fractures (canagliflozin)

GLP-1 Receptor Agonists (dulaglutide, exenatide, liraglutide, lixisenatide, semaglutide)

A1C reduction: 1.0-2.0%
Hypoglycemia: no, except when also receiving insulin or a sulfonylurea
Weight change: significant weight loss (6-10 kg); subcutaneous semaglutide *(Wegovy)* and subcutaneous liraglutide *(Saxenda)* also approved for chronic weight management
CV outcomes: reduced risk of MACE (dulaglutide, liraglutide, subcutaneous semaglutide)
Renal outcomes: reduced albuminuria (dulaglutide, liraglutide, subcutaneous semaglutide)
Renal: exenatide, lixisenatide: avoid with eGFR <30 mL/min/1.73 m^2; no dosage adjustments required for dulaglutide, liraglutide, semaglutide

Continued on next page

Table 3. Drugs for Type 2 Diabetes (continued)

GLP-1 Receptor Agonists (dulaglutide, exenatide, liraglutide, lixisenatide, semaglutide) (continued)

Adverse effects: GI (nausea, vomiting, diarrhea), injection-site reactions, renal impairment and acute renal failure, possible risk of pancreatitis, thyroid C-cell tumors reported in animals; contraindicated in patients with a personal or family history of multiple endocrine neoplasia type 2 (all except immediate-release exenatide and lixisenatide)

GIP/GLP-1 receptor agonist (tirzepatide)

A1C reduction: 2.0-2.5%
Hypoglycemia: no, except when also receiving insulin or a sulfonylurea
Weight change: significant weight loss (7-13 kg)
CV or renal outcomes: not yet determined
Renal: no dosage adjustment required
Adverse effects: GI (nausea, vomiting, diarrhea, abdominal pain), possible risk of pancreatitis, acute gall bladder disease, acute renal failure, increases in heart rate, thyroid C-cell tumors reported in animals; contraindicated in patients with a personal or family history of multiple endocrine neoplasia type 2

DPP-4 Inhibitors (alogliptin, linagliptin, saxagliptin, sitagliptin)

A1C reduction: 0.5-1.0%
Hypoglycemia: no, except when also receiving insulin or a sulfonylurea
Weight change: neutral
CV or renal outcomes: no benefit
Renal: dosage adjustment required (except linagliptin)
Adverse effects: possible risk of pancreatitis, joint pain, fatal hepatic failure; possible worsening HF with alogliptin, saxagliptin

Sulfonylureas (glimepiride, glipizide, glyburide)

A1C reduction: 1.0-1.5%
Hypoglycemia: yes
Weight change: gain
CV or renal outcomes: no benefit
Renal: dosage adjustments may be needed with glipizide and glimepiride
Adverse effects: many experts no longer use glyburide because of its adverse effects

CKD = chronic kidney disease; CV = cardiovascular; HF = heart failure; MACE = major adverse cardiovascular events

Continued on next page

Table 3. Drugs for Type 2 Diabetes (continued)
Thiazolidinedione (pioglitazone)
A1C reduction: 1.0-1.5%
Hypoglycemia: no, except when also receiving insulin or a sulfonylurea
Weight change: gain
CV outcomes: possibly reduced risk of MACE (also benefit in nonalcoholic steatohepatitis)
Renal outcomes: none
Renal: no dosage adjustment required
Adverse effects: possible risk of pancreatitis, macular edema, possible risk of bladder cancer, risk of bone fractures, increased risk of HF (contraindicated in patients with NYHA class III or IV HF)
CV = cardiovascular; HF = heart failure; MACE = major adverse cardiovascular events

DPP-4 INHIBITORS — The dipeptidyl peptidase-4 inhibitors alogliptin, linagliptin, saxagliptin, and sitagliptin potentiate glucose-dependent secretion of insulin and suppress glucagon secretion.[32-35] DPP-4 inhibitors have not increased or decreased the risk of MACE, hospitalization for HF, or progression of CKD in large randomized trials in patients with type 2 diabetes who have established CVD or are at high risk for CVD.[36]

SULFONYLUREAS — Sulfonylureas interact with ATP-sensitive potassium channels in the beta-cell membrane to increase secretion of insulin independent of nutrient intake. The sulfonylureas glimepiride, glipizide, and glyburide reduce A1C by 1-1.5%. Their effectiveness in reducing A1C, ease of use, and low cost led to their wide use as second-line agents, but they cause weight gain and hypoglycemia and have not been shown to have a beneficial effect on CV or renal outcomes.[37,38]

THIAZOLIDINEDIONES (TZDs) — Pioglitazone and rosiglitazone (not currently available in the US) increase the insulin sensitivity of adipose tissue, skeletal muscle, and the liver, and reduce hepatic glucose production. They reduce A1C by 1-1.5% but whether their benefits outweigh their risks (weight gain, HF, anemia, increased fracture risk) remains unclear. TZDs have been associated with an increased risk of HF and their labels contain a boxed warning stating that they can cause or exacerbate HF in some patients.[39] Pioglitazone has more beneficial effects on lipids than rosiglitazone.

MEGLITINIDES — Nateglinide and repaglinide, although structurally different from the sulfonylureas, also bind to ATP-sensitive potassium channels on beta cells and increase insulin release. Repaglinide is more effective than nateglinide in reducing A1C (1.0% vs 0.5%) and is safe for use in patients with CKD. Both drugs are rapidly absorbed and cleared; plasma levels of insulin peak 30-60 minutes after each dose and multiple daily doses are required. These drugs permit more dosing flexibility than sulfonylureas, but they can also cause hypoglycemia and have not been shown to have a beneficial effect on CV outcomes or to reduce microvascular complications.

ALPHA-GLUCOSIDASE INHIBITORS — Acarbose and miglitol inhibit the alpha-glucosidase enzymes that line the brush border of the small intestine, interfering with hydrolysis of carbohydrates and delaying absorption of glucose and other monosaccharides. To decrease postprandial glucose concentrations, acarbose and miglitol must be taken with each meal. Gastrointestinal adverse effects (e.g., bloating and flatulence) and minimal efficacy in reducing A1C limit use of these drugs.

PREGNANCY AND LACTATION — Metformin and (less so) glyburide appear to be relatively safe for use in pregnant women, but insulin is the drug of choice for treatment of type 2 diabetes in pregnant women because it does not cross the placenta. Data on the safety of other antihyperglycemic drugs during pregnancy remain insufficient to recommend their use.

Insulin and metformin are generally considered safe for use while breastfeeding. No adequate data are available on use of SGLT2 inhibitors, GLP-1 receptor agonists, or DPP-4 inhibitors in lactating women or their effects on the breastfed infant or milk production.

Table 4. Dosage and Cost of Antihyperglycemic Drugs

Drug	Some Formulations
Biguanide	
Metformin[3] – generic	500, 850, 1000 mg tabs
Riomet (Sun)	500 mg/5 mL soln (4, 16 oz)
extended-release – generic	500, 750, 1000 mg ER tabs
Glumetza (Santarus)	500, 1000 mg ER tabs
Riomet ER (Sun)	500 mg/5 mL soln (4, 16 oz)
SGLT2 Inhibitors	
Canagliflozin – *Invokana* (Janssen)	100, 300 mg tabs
Dapagliflozin – *Farxiga* (AstraZeneca)	5, 10 mg tabs
Empagliflozin – *Jardiance* (Boehringer Ingelheim/Lilly)	10, 25 mg tabs
Ertugliflozin – *Steglatro* (Merck)	5, 15 mg tabs
GLP-1 Receptor Agonists	
Dulaglutide – *Trulicity* (Lilly)[15]	0.75, 1.5, 3, 4.5 mg/0.5 mL single-dose pens
Exenatide – *Byetta* (AstraZeneca)	250 mcg/mL (1.2, 2.4 mL) prefilled pens
extended-release – *Bydureon BCise*[15]	2 mg/0.85 mL single-dose autoinjectors[19]
Liraglutide[20] – *Victoza* (Novo Nordisk)[15]	6 mg/mL (3 mL) prefilled pens
Lixisenatide – *Adlyxin* (Sanofi)	50, 100 mcg/mL (3 mL) prefilled pens

ER = extended release; SC = subcutaneous; soln = solution
1. Dosage for treatment of type 2 diabetes.
2. Approximate WAC for 4 weeks' or 30 days' treatment with the lowest usual adult dosage. WAC = wholesaler acquisition cost or manufacturer's published price to wholesalers; WAC represents a published catalogue or list price and may not represent an actual transactional price. Source: AnalySource® Monthly. October 5, 2022. Reprinted with permission by First Databank, Inc. All rights reserved. ©2022. www.fdbhealth.com/policies/drug-pricing-policy.
3. Metformin is contraindicated for use in patients with an eGFR <30 mL/min/1.73 m². Starting metformin in patients with an eGFR of 30-45 mL/min/1.73 m² is not recommended. If the eGFR falls below 45 mL/min/1.73 m² in patients already taking metformin, the benefits and risks of continuing the drug should be assessed.
4. Taken with meals.
5. Cost of one 16-ounce bottle.
6. Taken with the evening meal.
7. Tablets should be swallowed whole and not split, crushed, or chewed.
8. Taken with breakfast or the first meal of the day.
9. Maximum dose is 100 mg in patients with an eGFR of 30-<60 mL/min/1.73 m². Should not be started in patients with an eGFR <30 mL/min/1.73 m², however patients with albuminuria >300 mg/day can continue canagliflozin 100 mg once/day.

Usual Adult Dosage[1]	Cost[2]
1500-2550 mg/day PO divided bid-tid[4]	$2.70
	665.20[5]
1500-2000 mg PO once/day[6,7]	8.10
	4884.30
	599.00[5]
100-300 mg PO once/day[8-11]	570.10
5-10 mg PO once/day[10,12,13]	548.80
10-25 mg PO once/day[10-12]	570.50
5-15 mg PO once/day[10,12,14]	324.60
0.75 or 1.5 mg SC once/week[16]	886.60
5 or 10 mcg SC bid[17,18]	801.20
2 mg SC once/week[18]	780.00
1.2 or 1.8 mg SC once/day[21]	709.60
20 mcg SC once/day[22]	678.50

10. Contraindicated in patients on dialysis.
11. Not recommended to improve glycemic control in patients with type 2 diabetes and an eGFR <30 mL/min/1.73 m².
12. Taken in the morning, with or without food.
14. Not recommended in patients with an eGFR <45 mL/min/1.73 m².
15. Contraindicated in patients with a personal or family history of medullary thyroid carcinoma and in patients with multiple endocrine neoplasia syndrome type 2.
16. Dose can be increased after at least 4 weeks on previous dose.
17. Starting dosage is 5 mcg twice daily, up to an hour before morning and evening meals. After one month, the dosage can be increased to 10 mcg twice daily.
18. The immediate-release formulation is not recommended in patients with a CrCl <30 mL/min and the extended-release formulation is not recommended in those with an eGFR <45 mL/min/1.73 m².
19. Must be reconstituted before administration.
20. Liraglutide is approved as *Saxenda* and semaglutide as *Wegovy* for chronic weight management in patients with and without type 2 diabetes.
21. Starting dosage is 0.6 mg once daily for 7 days, followed by 1.2 mg thereafter. The dose can be increased after at least one week on previous dose.
22. Starting dosage is 10 mcg once daily, up to an hour before the morning meal, for 14 days, followed by 20 mcg thereafter.

Continued on next page

Drugs for Type 2 Diabetes

Table 4. Dosage and Cost of Antihyperglycemic Drugs (continued)	
Drug	**Some Formulations**
GLP-1 Receptor Agonists (continued)	
Semaglutide[20] – *Ozempic* (Novo Nordisk)[15]	0.68, 1.34, 2.68 mg/mL (1.5 mL, 3 mL) prefilled pens
Rybelsus (Novo Nordisk)[15]	3, 7, 14 mg tabs
GIP/GLP-1 Receptor Agonist	
Tirzepatide – *Mounjaro* (Lilly)[15]	2.5, 5, 7.5, 10, 12.5, 15 mg/0.5 mL single-dose pens
DPP-4 Inhibitors	
Alogliptin – generic *Nesina* (Takeda)	6.25, 12.5, 25 mg tabs
Linagliptin – *Tradjenta* (Boehringer Ingelheim)	5 mg tabs
Saxagliptin – *Onglyza* (AstraZeneca)	2.5, 5 mg tabs
Sitagliptin – *Januvia* (Merck)	25, 50, 100 mg tabs
Sulfonylureas	
Glimepiride – generic *Amaryl* (Sanofi)	1, 2, 4 mg tabs
Glipizide – generic extended-release – generic *Glucotrol XL*	5, 10 mg tabs 2.5, 5, 10 mg ER tabs 10 mg ER tabs
Glyburide[31] – generic micronized tablets – generic *Glynase Prestab* (Pfizer)	1.25, 2.5, 5 mg tabs 1.5, 3, 6 mg tabs
Thiazolidinedione	
Pioglitazone – generic *Actos* (Takeda)	15, 30, 45 mg tabs

ER = extended release; SC = subcutaneous

23. Starting dosage is 0.25 mg once weekly for 4 weeks, followed by 0.5 mg once weekly. The dose can be increased after at least 4 weeks on previous dose.
24. Starting dosage is 3 mg once daily for 30 days. Dose can be increased after at least 4 weeks on previous dose. Tablets should be swallowed whole with no more than 4 ounces of water 30 minutes before first food, drink, or other oral drugs.
25. Starting dosage is 2.5 mg once weekly for 4 weeks, followed by 5 mg once weekly. The dose can be increased in 2.5-mg increments once weekly as needed.
26. The recommended dosage is 12.5 mg once daily in patients with a CrCl of 30-59 mL/min and 6.25 mg once daily in those with a CrCl <30 mL/min.
27. The recommended dosage is 2.5 mg once daily in patients with an eGFR <45 mL/min/1.73 m^2.

Usual Adult Dosage[1]	Cost[2]
0.5-2 mg SC once/week[23]	$892.10
7 or 14 PO mg once/day[24]	892.10
5-15 mg SC once/week[25]	974.30
25 mg PO once/day[26]	195.00
	409.00
5 mg PO once/day	504.90
5 mg PO once/day[27]	471.00
100 mg PO once/day[28]	521.40
1-4 mg PO once/day[8,29]	2.70
	39.90
10-20 mg PO once/day[8] or divided bid[30]	2.00
5-20 mg PO once/day[7,8]	5.10
	21.30
1.25-20 mg PO once/day[8] or divided bid[4]	1.80
0.75-12 mg PO once/day[8] or divided bid[4]	5.00
	28.00
15-45 mg PO once/day[32,33]	4.00
	388.60

28. The recommended dosage is 50 mg once daily in patients with an eGFR of 30-<45 mL/min/1.73 m^2 and 25 mg once daily in those with an eGFR <30 mL/min/1.73 m^2.
29. Dose can be increased in 1- or 2-mg increments no more frequently than every 1-2 weeks to a maximum of 8 mg once daily.
30. Doses >15 mg/day should be divided and given before meals of adequate caloric content.
31. Because of its adverse effects, many experts no longer recommend use of glyburide (MC Riddle. J Clin Endocrinol Metab 2010; 95:4867).
32. Should not be started in patients with ALT >3 times upper limit of normal (ULN) with serum total bilirubin >2 times ULN or in those with active bladder cancer. Contraindicated in patients with NYHA class III or IV heart failure.
33. The starting dosage of pioglitazone is 15 mg once daily in patients with NYHA class I or II heart failure.

Continued on next page

Table 4. Dosage and Cost of Antihyperglycemic Drugs (continued)	
Drug	**Some Formulations**
Meglitinides	
Nateglinide – generic	60, 120 mg tabs
Repaglinide – generic	0.5, 1, 2 mg tabs
Alpha-Glucosidase Inhibitors	
Acarbose – generic	25, 50, 100 mg tabs
Miglitol – generic	25, 50, 100 mg tabs
Metformin Combination Products	
Metformin/glipizide[3] – generic	250/2.5, 500/2.5, 500/5 mg tabs
Metformin/glyburide[3,31] – generic	250/1.25, 500/2.5, 500/5 mg tabs
Metformin/pioglitazone[3] – generic *Actoplus Met* (Takeda)	500/15, 850/15 mg tabs 800/15 mg tabs
Metformin/alogliptin[3] – generic *Kazano* (Takeda)	500/12.5, 1000/12.5 mg tabs

Metformin/linagliptin[3] – *Jentadueto*
  (Boehringer Ingelheim)
  Jentadueto XR
	500/2.5, 850/2.5, 1000/2.5 mg
	  tabs
	1000/2.5, 1000/5 mg ER tabs

Metformin/saxagliptin[3] – *Kombiglyze XR*
  (BMS)
	500/5, 1000/2.5, 1000/5 mg
	  ER tabs

Metformin/sitagliptin[3] – *Janumet* (Merck)
  Janumet XR
	500/50, 1000/50 mg tabs
	500/50, 1000/50, 1000/100 mg
	  ER tabs

Metformin/canagliflozin[3]– *Invokamet*
  (Janssen)
  Invokamet XR
	500/50, 1000/50, 500/150,
	  1000/150 mg tabs
	500/50, 1000/50, 500/150,
	  1000/150 mg ER tabs

Metformin/dapagliflozin[3] – *Xigduo XR*
  (AstraZeneca)
	1000/2.5, 500/5, 1000/5,
	  500/10, 1000/10 mg ER tabs

Metformin/empagliflozin[3] – *Synjardy*
  (Boehringer Ingelheim/Lilly)
  Synjardy XR
	500/5, 1000/5, 500/12.5,
	  1000/12.5 mg tabs
	1000/5, 1000/10, 1000/12.5,
	  1000/25 mg ER tabs

ER = extended release
34. Taken 15-30 minutes before meals. Should not be taken if meal is missed.
35. A starting dose of 0.5 mg tid with meals is recommended for patients with a CrCl of 20-40 mL/min.
36. Not recommended for patients with a serum creatinine >2 mg/dL or a CrCl <25 mL/min/1.73 m².
37. Not recommended in patients with a CrCl <25 mL/min.
38. Patients who need 2000 mg/day of metformin should take two 1000/2.5 mg tablets once daily.

Usual Adult Dosage[1]	Cost[2]
60-120 mg PO tid[34]	$44.90
1-4 mg PO tid[34,35]	18.00
50-100 mg PO tid[4,36]	41.30
50-100 mg PO tid[4,37]	291.40
500/2.5 mg PO bid[4]	31.20
500/5 mg PO bid[4]	35.20
500/15 mg PO bid[4,32]	75.00
	590.40
1000/12.5 mg PO bid[4,14]	195.00
	409.00
500/2.5-1000/2.5 mg PO bid[4]	436.20
1000/5-2000/5 mg PO once/day[4,7,38]	504.90
1000/5-2000/5 mg PO once/day[6,7]	471.00
500/50-1000/50 mg PO bid[4]	521.40
1000/100-2000/100 mg PO once/day[6,7]	521.40
500/50-500/150 mg PO bid[4,39]	570.10
1000/100-1000/300 mg PO once/day[7,8,39]	570.10
500/5-1000/10 mg PO once/day[7,8,38,40]	548.80
500/5-1000/12.5 mg PO bid[4,40]	570.50
1000/5-1000/25 mg PO once/day[7,8,40]	285.20

39. Maximum daily dose is 2000/300 mg in patients with an eGFR ≥60 mL/min/1.73 m². Patients with an eGFR of 45-<60 mL/min/1.73 m² should not receive more than 50 mg of canagliflozin bid. Contraindicated in patients with an eGFR <30 mL/min/1.73 m², end-stage renal disease, or dialysis.
40. Contraindicated for use in patients with eGFR <30 mL/min/1.73 m², end-stage renal disease, or dialysis.

Continued on next page

Table 4. Dosage and Cost of Antihyperglycemic Drugs (continued)	
Drug	**Some Formulations**
Metformin Combination Products (continued)	
Metformin/ertugliflozin[3] – *Segluromet* (Merck)	500/2.5, 500/7.5, 1000/2.5, 1000/7.5 mg tabs
Other Combination Products	
Glimepiride/pioglitazone – generic *Duetact* (Takeda)	2/30, 4/30 mg tabs
Alogliptin/pioglitazone – generic *Oseni* (Takeda)	12.5/15, 12.5/30, 12.5/45, 25/15, 25/30, 25/45 mg tabs
Dapagliflozin/saxagliptin – *Qtern* (AstraZeneca)	5/5, 10/5 mg tabs
Empagliflozin/linagliptin – *Glyxambi* (Boehringer Ingelheim/Lilly)	10/5, 25/5 mg tabs
Ertugliflozin/sitagliptin – *Steglujan* (Merck)	5/100, 15/100 mg tabs
Long-Acting Insulin/GLP-1 Receptor Agonist Combinations	
Insulin degludec/liraglutide[15] – *Xultophy* 100/3.6 (Novo Nordisk)	3 mL prefilled pens[44]
Insulin glargine/lixisenatide – *Soliqua* 100/33 (Sanofi)	3 mL prefilled pens[48]

SC = subcutaneous
41. The recommended dose of alogliptin is 12.5 mg/day in patients with a CrCl of 30-59 mL/min.
42. Starting dosage is 5 mg/5 mg in patients already taking dapagliflozin.
43. Contraindicated for use in patients with eGFR <45 mL/min/1.73 m², end-stage renal disease, or dialysis.
44. Contains 100 units/mL of insulin degludec and 3.6 mg/mL of liraglutide.
45. Should be given at the same time each day with or without food.
46. Basal insulin or a GLP-1 receptor agonist should be discontinued before starting treatment. Starting dosage is 10 units/0.36 mg in patients naive to basal insulin or a GLP-1 receptor agonist and is 16 units/0.58 mg in those on basal insulin or a GLP-1 receptor agonist; titrate up or down by 2 units every 3-4 days to achieve desired fasting plasma glucose.

Usual Adult Dosage[1]	Cost[2]
500/2.5-1000/7.5 mg PO bid[4,40]	$324.60
2/30-4/30 mg PO once/day[8,32,33]	390.50
	593.80
25/15-25/45 mg PO once/day[12,32,33,41]	195.00
	409.00
10/5 mg PO once/day[12,42,43]	548.80
10/5-25/5 mg PO once/day[10-12]	570.50
5/100-15/100 mg PO once/day[10,12,14]	549.90
16-50 units SC once/day[45,46]	943.80[47]
15-60 units SC once/day[49,50]	646.40[47]

47. Cost of 30 days' treatment for a patient using *Xultophy* 40 units/1.44 mg daily or *Soliqua* 40 units/13.3 mcg daily.
48. Contains 100 units/mL of insulin glargine and 33 mcg/mL of lixisenatide.
49. Within one hour before first meal of the day.
50. Basal insulin or a GLP-1 receptor agonist should be discontinued before starting treatment. Starting dosage is 15 units/5 mcg in patients naive to basal insulin or a GLP-1 receptor agonist, on <30 units of basal insulin, or on a GLP-1 receptor agonist, and is 30 units/10 mcg in those on 30-60 units of basal insulin; titrate up or down by 2-4 units/week to achieve desired fasting plasma glucose.

Table 5. Some Drug Interactions with Antihyperglycemic Drugs[1-3]

Biguanide (metformin)

- OCT1 inhibitors (e.g., codeine) or MATE inhibitors (e.g., cimetidine) can increase serum concentrations of metformin
- OCT1 inducers (e.g., metoprolol) can decrease serum concentrations of metformin
- Agents that cause lactic acidosis (e.g., alcohol, carbonic anhydrase inhibitors, iodinated contrast media) can increase the risk of metformin-induced lactic acidosis
- Increased risk of acute kidney injury with iodinated contrast media
- Decreased anticoagulant effect of warfarin; warfarin can increase the hypoglycemic effect of metformin

SGLT2 Inhibitors (canagliflozin, dapagliflozin, empagliflozin, ertugliflozin)

- Decreased serum concentrations of lithium

Canagliflozin:

- UGT inducers (e.g., rifampin, phenytoin, phenobarbital, ritonavir) can decrease canagliflozin exposure and possibly its efficacy
- Increased serum concentrations of digoxin

GLP-1 Receptor Agonists (dulaglutide, exenatide, liraglutide, lixisenatide, semaglutide)

- May decrease rate and extent of absorption of oral medications taken concomitantly

GIP/GLP-1 Receptor Agonists (tirzepatide)

- May decrease rate and extent of absorption of oral medications taken concomitantly

Continued on next page

1. American Diabetes Association. Introduction: standards of medical care in diabetes—2022. Diabetes Care 2022; 45(Suppl 1):S1.
2. Insulins for type 2 diabetes. Med Lett Drugs Ther 2019; 61:65.
3. FDA Drug Safety Communication: FDA revises warnings regarding use of the diabetes medicine metformin in certain patients with reduced kidney function. April 2017. Available at: https://bit.ly/3SdEFRN. Accessed October 27, 2022.
4. CL Roumie et al. Association of treatment with metformin vs sulfonylurea with major adverse cardiovascular events among patients with diabetes and reduced kidney function. JAMA 2019; 322:1167.
5. TL Richardson Jr et al. Hospitalization for heart failure among patients with diabetes mellitus and reduced kidney function treated with metformin versus sulfonylureas: a retrospective cohort study. J Am Heart Assoc 2021; 10:e019211.
6. PY Chu et al. Hospitalization for lactic acidosis among patients with reduced kidney function treated with metformin or sulfonylureas. Diabetes Care 2020; 43:1462.

Table 5. Some Drug Interactions with Antihyperglycemic Drugs[1-3] (continued)

DPP-4 Inhibitors (alogliptin, linagliptin, saxagliptin, sitagliptin)

▶ Can increase the risk of ACE inhibitor-associated angioedema

Linagliptin:

▶ Strong P-gp or CYP3A4 inducers can decrease linagliptin serum concentrations

Saxagliptin:

▶ Strong CYP3A4/5 inhibitors can increase saxagliptin serum concentrations; saxagliptin daily dose should not exceed 2.5 mg when used with a strong CYP3A4/5 inhibitor. CYP3A4 inducers can decrease efficacy of saxagliptin

Sitagliptin:

▶ May increase digoxin serum concentrations

Sulfonylureas (glimepiride, glipizide, glyburide)

▶ CYP2C9 inhibitors can increase serum concentration of sulfonylureas

▶ Increased risk of hepatotoxicity with bosentan; concurrent use is contraindicated

Thiazolidinediones (pioglitazone)

▶ Increased risk of osteoporosis and fracture with PPIs

▶ CYP2C8 inhibitors can increase and 2C8 inducers can decrease pioglitazone serum concentrations; pioglitazone daily dose should not exceed 15 mg when used with a strong 2C8 inhibitor

MATE = multidrug and toxin extruder; OCT1 = organic cation transporter 1; P-gp = P-glycoprotein; UGT = UDP-glucuronosyltransferase

1. The risk of hypoglycemia is increased when taken with other drugs that lower blood glucose.
2. Inhibitors and inducers of CYP enzymes, P-glycoprotein and other transporters. Med Lett Drugs Ther 2021 October 20 (epub). Available at: medicalletter.org/downloads/CYP_PGP_Tables.pdf.
3. M May and C Schindler. Clinically and pharmacologically relevant interactions of antidiabetic drugs. Ther Adv Endocrinol Metab 2016; 7:69.

7. TA Zelniker et al. Comparison of the effects of glucagon-like peptide receptor agonists and sodium-glucose cotransporter 2 inhibitors for prevention of major adverse cardiovascular and renal outcomes in type 2 diabetes mellitus. Circulation 2019; 139:2022.

8. The GRADE Study Research Group. Glycemia reduction in type 2 diabetes – glycemic outcomes. N Engl J Med 2022; 387:1063.

9. The GRADE Study Research Group. Glycemia reduction in type 2 diabetes – microvascular and cardiovascular outcomes. N Engl J Med 2022; 387:1075.

10. R Pratley et al. Oral semaglutide versus subcutaneous liraglutide and placebo in type 2 diabetes (PIONEER 4): a randomised, double-blind, phase 3a trial. Lancet 2019; 394:39.

11. VR Aroda et al. PIONEER 1: randomized clinical trial of the efficacy and safety of oral semaglutide monotherapy in comparison with placebo in patients with type 2 diabetes. Diabetes Care 2019; 42:1724.

12. HW Rodbard et al. Oral semaglutide versus empagliflozin in patients with type 2 diabetes uncontrolled on metformin: the PIONEER 2 trial. Diabetes Care 2019; 42:2272.

13. J Rosenstock et al. Effect of additional oral semaglutide vs sitagliptin on glycated hemoglobin in adults with type 2 diabetes uncontrolled with metformin alone or with sulfonylurea: the PIONEER 3 randomized clinical trial. JAMA 2019; 321:1466.
14. B Neal et al. Canagliflozin and cardiovascular and renal events in type 2 diabetes. N Engl J Med 2017; 377:644.
15. V Perkovic et al. Canagliflozin and renal outcomes in type 2 diabetes and nephropathy. N Engl J Med 2019; 380;2295.
16. SD Wiviott et al. Dapagliflozin and cardiovascular outcomes in type 2 diabetes. N Engl J Med 2019; 380:347.
17. SD Solomon et al. Dapagliflozin in heart failure with mildly reduced or preserved ejection fraction. N Engl J Med 2022; 387:1089.
18. HJL Heerspink et al. Dapagliflozin in patients with chronic kidney disease. N Engl J Med 2020; 383:1436.
19. M Packer et al. Cardiovascular and renal outcomes with empagliflozin in heart failure. N Engl J Med 2020; 383:1413.
20. SD Anker et al. Empagliflozin in heart failure with a preserved ejection fraction. N Engl J Med 2021; 385:1451.
21. CP Cannon et al. Cardiovascular outcomes with ertugliflozin in type 2 diabetes. N Engl J Med 2020; 383:1425.
22. HC Gerstein et al. Dulaglutide and cardiovascular outcomes in type 2 diabetes (REWIND): a double-blind, randomised placebo-controlled trial. Lancet 2019; 394:121.
23. HC Gerstein et al. Dulaglutide and renal outcomes in type 2 diabetes: an exploratory analysis of the REWIND randomised, placebo-controlled trial. Lancet 2019; 394:131.
24. SP Marso et al. Liraglutide and cardiovascular outcomes in type 2 diabetes. N Engl J Med 2016; 375:311.
25. JFE Mann et al. Liraglutide and renal outcomes in type 2 diabetes. N Engl J Med 2017; 377:839.
26. SP Marso et al. Semaglutide and cardiovascular outcomes in patients with type 2 diabetes. N Engl J Med 2016; 375:1834.
27. Semaglutide (Ozempic) – another injectable GLP-1 receptor agonist for type 2 diabetes. Med Lett Drugs Ther 2018; 60:19.
28. Lixisenatide for type 2 diabetes. Med Lett Drugs Ther 2017; 59:19.
29. RR Holman et al. Effects of once-weekly exenatide on cardiovascular outcomes in type 2 diabetes. N Engl J Med 2017; 377:1228.
30. MA Pfeffer et al. Lixisenatide in patients with type 2 diabetes and acute coronary syndrome. N Engl J Med 2015; 373:2247.
31. Tirzepatide (Mounjaro) for type 2 diabetes Med Lett Drugs Ther 2022; 64:105.
32. Alogliptin (Nesina) for type 2 diabetes. Med Lett Drugs Ther 2013; 55:41.
33. Linagliptin (Tradjenta) – a new DPP-4 inhibitor for type 2 diabetes. Med Lett Drugs Ther 2011; 53:49.
34. Saxagliptin (Onglyza) for type 2 diabetes. Med Lett Drugs Ther 2009; 51:85.
35. Sitagliptin (Januvia) for type 2 diabetes. Med Lett Drugs Ther 2007; 49:1.
36. J Rosenstock et al. Effect of linagliptin vs placebo on major cardiovascular outcomes in adults with type 2 diabetes and high cardiovascular and renal risk: the CARMELINA randomized clinical trial. JAMA 2019; 321:69.

37. KB Filion et al. Sulfonylureas as initial treatment for type 2 diabetes and the risk of adverse cardiovascular events: a population-based cohort study. Br J Clin Pharmacol 2019; 85:2378.
38. A Douros et al. Sulfonylureas as second line drugs in type 2 diabetes and the risk of cardiovascular and hypoglycaemic events: population based cohort study BMJ 2018; 362:k2693.
39. AV Hernandez et al. Thiazolidinediones and risk of heart failure in patients with or at high risk of type 2 diabetes mellitus: a meta-analysis and meta-regression analysis of placebo-controlled randomized clinical trials. Am J Cardiovasc Drugs 2011; 11:115.

DRUGS FOR
GERD and Peptic Ulcer Disease

Original publication date – April 2022 (revised December 2022)

GASTROESOPHAGEAL REFLUX DISEASE

Gastroesophageal reflux disease (GERD) is the most common GI condition encountered in the outpatient setting; it affects about 20% of people in the US.

DIAGNOSIS — Heartburn and regurgitation are the classic symptoms of GERD. Other symptoms include dyspepsia, chest pain, belching, and chronic cough. Endoscopy is recommended to evaluate alarm signs and symptoms such as dysphagia, GI bleeding, anemia, weight loss, and persistent vomiting. It is also recommended for patients at high risk for complications, including those whose symptoms do not respond adequately to acid suppression, and for those with multiple risk factors for Barrett's esophagus.[1,2]

LIFESTYLE MODIFICATION — Lifestyle modifications, such as tobacco cessation, not lying down for at least 2 hours after eating or drinking, and elevating the head of the bed, should be a component of GERD management.[3] Weight loss can improve symptoms in patients who are overweight or have recently gained weight.[4,5] Routine avoidance of foods that have been associated with reflux, such as chocolate, caffeine, alcohol, and spicy foods, may be helpful, especially for nocturnal symptoms, but is generally not necessary.[2]

Key Points: Drugs for GERD and PUD
GERD
▸ Lifestyle modifications, such as not lying down for at least 2 hours after eating or drinking, elevating the head of the bed, and weight loss in patients who are overweight or have recently gained weight, should be a component of management.
▸ As-needed use of an antacid or H2-receptor antagonist (H2RA) is recommended for patients with infrequent or mild symptoms.
▸ Daily use of a proton pump inhibitor (PPI) is recommended for patients with more frequent or severe symptoms or erosive esophagitis.
▸ PPIs are more effective than H2RAs in relieving chronic heartburn and regurgitation and in healing erosive esophagitis.
▸ Addition of an H2RA as needed may be beneficial for patients who have symptoms despite twice-daily PPI treatment.
PUD
▸ *Helicobacter pylori* infection and use of nonsteroidal anti-inflammatory drugs cause most cases of PUD.
▸ All patients with PUD should be tested for *H. pylori*.
▸ All patients with PUD should be treated with a PPI.
▸ If the underlying cause of PUD can be identified and eliminated, long-term PPI therapy may not be needed.
▸ Bismuth quadruple therapy is recommended for first-line treatment of *H. pylori* infection; rifabutin triple therapy is an alternative.
▸ Clarithromycin-based therapy should only be used when antimicrobial susceptibility tests have shown that *H. pylori* is susceptible to clarithromycin or in areas where *H. pylori* resistance to clarithromycin is known to be <15%.
▸ All patients should be tested for eradication of *H. pylori* ≥4 weeks after completion of therapy.

CHOICE OF DRUGS — Drugs that suppress gastric acid are the standard treatment for GERD (see Table 2). The choice of drug depends on the frequency and severity of symptoms and the presence or absence of erosive esophagitis. Patients with infrequent or mild symptoms can be treated with an antacid or H2-receptor antagonist (H2RA) as needed. For patients whose symptoms are inadequately controlled on these agents and those with more frequent or severe symptoms or erosive esophagitis, a proton pump inhibitor (PPI) is recommended. PPIs decrease GERD symptoms and heal esophagitis more effectively than H2RAs and are generally preferred.

ANTACIDS — Antacids containing aluminum, magnesium, and/or calcium carbonate can provide rapid but transient relief of GERD symptoms.

Adverse Effects – Aluminum and calcium carbonate can cause constipation, and magnesium-based antacids can cause diarrhea.

Drug Interactions – Antacids can decrease the absorption of some other drugs (e.g., tetracyclines, levofloxacin) by altering gastric acidity or by binding to other drugs in the GI tract.

Pregnancy – Heartburn occurs commonly during pregnancy; it is largely attributed to a progesterone-mediated decrease in lower esophageal sphincter tone. Antacids can be tried for symptomatic relief, but products containing sodium bicarbonate (may cause metabolic alkalosis and fluid overload) or magnesium trisilicate (long-term use of high doses has been associated with nephrolithiasis, hypotonia, and respiratory distress in the fetus) should be avoided.[6]

H2-RECEPTOR ANTAGONISTS — H2RAs inhibit the action of histamine at H2 receptors on parietal cells, decreasing basal acid secretion and, to a much lesser extent, food-stimulated acid secretion. H2RAs have a faster onset of action than PPIs, but they are less effective in relieving chronic heartburn and regurgitation and in healing erosive esophagitis,[2] and tolerance can develop quickly with continuous use.

Adverse Effects – Severe adverse effects are uncommon with H2RAs. Hepatic enzyme elevations, hematologic toxicity, and CNS effects such as headache, lethargy, depression, and cognitive impairment have occurred. Cimetidine is weakly antiandrogenic; chronic use may rarely cause reversible impotence and gynecomastia. The FDA has withdrawn all prescription and OTC formulations of ranitidine because they may contain the carcinogen *N*-nitrosodimethylamine (NDMA).

Drug Interactions – H2RAs can decrease serum concentrations of drugs that require gastric acidity for absorption, such as itraconazole and the antiretroviral drugs rilpivirine and atazanavir. Cimetidine is a moderate inhibitor of CYP1A2, 2C19, and 2D6; it can increase serum concentrations of drugs that are metabolized by these enzymes, such warfarin and fluoxetine.[7] Famotidine and nizatidine are less likely to affect the hepatic metabolism of other drugs.

Pregnancy – H2RAs are generally considered safe for use during pregnancy, but adequate studies are lacking.

PROTON PUMP INHIBITORS — PPIs bind to the activated proton pump on the apical membrane of parietal cells, resulting in variably potent inhibition of acid secretion into the gastric lumen (see Table 1). They are more effective than H2RAs in relieving chronic heartburn and regurgitation and in healing erosive esophagitis. Treatment with a PPI for 8 weeks is recommended for healing of erosive esophagitis.[2] Almost all patients with erosive esophagitis will have a relapse of symptoms within 6 months of stopping the PPI and most will require long-term maintenance therapy.

PPIs have short serum half-lives, but their duration of action is longer than that of H2RAs, allowing for once-daily dosing in most patients with GERD. For patients who continue to have symptoms, switching to twice-daily dosing is more effective than increasing the dose.[8] Addition of an H2RA as needed may be helpful for patients who still have symptoms despite twice-daily PPI treatment.

PPIs generally are most effective when taken on an empty stomach, 30-60 minutes before a meal. Dexlansoprazole can be taken without regard to meals. Other antisecretory drugs such as H2RAs should not be taken at the same time as a PPI. Unlike H2RAs, tolerance to PPIs does not develop with continuous use.

Adverse Effects – Short-term use of PPIs is generally well tolerated. Headache, nausea, abdominal pain, constipation, flatulence, and diarrhea can occur. Gynecomastia, hepatic failure, subacute myopathy, arthralgia, severe rash, lupus erythematosus, and acute interstitial nephritis have been reported.

Table 1. Relative Potency of PPIs[1]	
Drug	Omeprazole Equivalent
Pantoprazole 20 mg	4.5 mg
Lansoprazole 15 mg	13.5 mg
Omeprazole 20 mg	20 mg
Esomeprazole 20 mg	32 mg
Rabeprazole 20 mg	36 mg
Dexlansoprazole 30 mg[2]	50-60 mg

1. Based on the percentage time gastric pH is >4 over a 24-hour period with once-daily dosing. Adapted from DY Graham and A Tansel. Clin Gastroenterol Hepatol 2018; 16:800.
2. Compared to twice-daily use of other PPIs, once-daily dexlansoprazole is less "potent".

In observational studies, long-term PPI use has been associated with a number of safety concerns, including dementia, vitamin B12 deficiency, chronic kidney disease, and increased all-cause mortality.[9,10] Most of these concerns are not supported by a causal mechanism or consistent data. The FDA has issued safety warnings about an association between long-term PPI use and hypomagnesemia, increased fracture risk, and *Clostridioides difficile* infection. In a population-based cohort study in new users of PPIs and H2RAs, use of PPIs was associated with a 45% greater risk of gastric cancer, but the absolute risk was low.[11] The benefits of PPI treatment generally outweigh the risks in patients with a clear indication for long-term treatment.[12]

Drug Interactions – PPIs may decrease serum concentrations of drugs that require gastric acidity for absorption, such as itraconazole and the antiretroviral drugs rilpivirine and atazanavir.

Most PPIs are metabolized primarily by CYP2C19. Patients who are CYP2C19 ultra-rapid metabolizers may have a decreased response to PPI treatment, and poor metabolizers (many Asian patients) may have higher PPI serum concentrations.[13] Lansoprazole and dexlansoprazole are metabolized primarily by CYP3A4. Omeprazole and esomeprazole are moderate inhibitors of CYP2C19 and could increase serum concentrations of drugs metabolized by this pathway, such as warfarin and phenytoin.[7,14]

Table 2. Some Oral Drugs for GERD and PUD

Drug	Some Available Oral Formulations
H2-Receptor Antagonists (H2RAs)[3]	
Cimetidine – generic	200, 300, 400, 800 mg tabs; 300 mg/5 mL soln
Tagamet HB (OTC)[5] (Medtech)	200 mg tabs
Famotidine[6] – generic	20, 40 mg tabs; 40 mg/5 mL susp
Pepcid AC (OTC)[5] (J&J Consumer)	10, 20 mg tabs
Zantac 360 (OTC)[5] (Sanofi)	10, 20 mg tabs
Nizatidine – generic	150, 300 mg caps; 15 mg/mL soln
Proton Pump Inhibitors (PPIs)[8]	
Dexlansoprazole – generic	30, 60 mg delayed-release caps[9]
Dexilant (Takeda)	
Esomeprazole magnesium[10] – generic	20, 40 mg delayed-release caps[9]
Nexium (AstraZeneca)	20, 40 mg delayed-release caps[9]; 2.5, 5, 10, 20, 40 mg powder for delayed-release susp
Nexium 24HR (OTC)[5] (GSK)	20 mg delayed-release caps, tabs
Lansoprazole – generic	15, 30 mg delayed-release caps[9]; 15, 30 mg ODTs
Prevacid (Takeda)	30 mg delayed-release caps
Prevacid 24HR (OTC)[5] (Perrigo)	15 mg delayed-release caps
Omeprazole[12] – generic	10, 20, 40 mg delayed-release caps[9]
Prilosec (Covis)	2.5, 10 mg powder for delayed-release susp
Prilosec OTC[5] (P&G)	20 mg delayed-release tabs

ODTs = orally disintegrating tablets; OTC = over the counter; soln = solution; susp = suspension

1. The lower end of the range is generally used for initial treatment of GERD. Higher or more frequent doses may be needed for patients with erosive esophagitis, peptic ulcer disease, hypersecretory conditions such as Zollinger-Ellison syndrome, or for treatment of _H. pylori_ infection. Dosage adjustments may be needed for renal or hepatic impairment.
2. Approximate WAC for 30 days' treatment with the lowest usual adult dosage. WAC = wholesaler acquisition cost or manufacturer's published price to wholesalers; WAC represents a published catalogue or list price and may not represent an actual transactional price. Source: AnalySource® Monthly. March 5, 2022. Reprinted with permission by First Databank, Inc. All rights reserved. ©2022. www.fdbhealth.com/policies/drug-pricing-policy.
3. In April 2020, the FDA requested that all OTC and prescription ranitidine products be removed from the market because they may contain the carcinogen _N_-nitrosodimethylamine (NDMA).
4. Taking the total daily dose in the evening may also be effective.

Usual Adult Dosage[1]	Cost[2]
200-400 mg PO bid[4]	$7.80
	16.30
20-40 mg PO bid[4]	6.00
	15.40[7]
	12.10[7]
150 mg PO bid[4]	72.30
30-60 mg PO once/day	262.10
	308.40
20-40 mg PO once/day	15.30
	275.30
	16.40[11]
15-30 mg PO once/day	16.10
	414.90
	18.50[11]
20-40 mg PO once/day	16.20
	830.30
	16.80[11]

5. May also be available generically. Not FDA-approved for use in GERD or peptic ulcer disease.
6. Also available in combination with ibuprofen (Duexis).
7. Approximate WAC for fifty 20-mg tablets.
8. PPIs are generally taken 30-60 minutes before the first meal of the day. Taking one dose before the evening meal or taking the drug twice daily may be more effective for nocturnal acid control. PPIs should generally be swallowed whole and should not be crushed or chewed. Dexlansoprazole can be taken with or without food. Omeprazole/sodium bicarbonate should be taken on an empty stomach at least 1 hour before a meal.
9. Capsules can be opened and their contents sprinkled on soft food such as applesauce and consumed immediately.
10. Also available in combination with naproxen (Vimovo, and generics).
11. Approximate WAC for 28 capsules or tablets.
12. Also available in combination with amoxicillin/clarithromycin (Omeclamox-Pak).

Continued on next page

Table 2. Some Oral Drugs for GERD and PUD (continued)	
Drug	**Some Available Oral Formulations**
Proton Pump Inhibitors (PPIs)[8] (continued)	
Omeprazole/sodium bicarbonate[13] – generic	20/1680, 40/1680 mg/packets for susp; 20 mg/1.1 g, 40 mg/1.1 g caps[14]
Zegerid (Bausch)	
Zegerid OTC[5] (Bayer)	20 mg/1.1 g, 40 mg/1.1 g caps[14]
Pantoprazole – generic	20, 40 mg delayed-release tabs
Protonix (Pfizer)	20, 40 mg delayed-release tabs; 40 mg delayed-release granules for susp
Rabeprazole – generic	20 mg delayed-release tabs
Aciphex (Woodward)	
Aciphex Sprinkle	5, 10 mg delayed-release sprinkle caps[15]
Others	
Misoprostol[16,17] – generic	100, 200 mcg tabs
Cytotec (Pfizer)	
Sucralfate[18] – generic	1 g tabs; 1 g/10 mL susp
Carafate (Abbvie)	

OTC = over the counter; susp = suspension
13. Immediate-release formulation of omeprazole. Should be used with caution in patients on a low-sodium diet.
14. Since each capsule contains 1.1 g of sodium bicarbonate, two 20-mg capsules are not equivalent to one 40-mg capsule.

The antiplatelet drug clopidogrel (*Plavix*, and generics) is converted to its active form by CYP2C19; inhibition of CYP2C19 may interfere with its activation. Whether concurrent use of clopidogrel and a PPI results in clinically significant adverse cardiovascular outcomes is not clear.[15,16] Since omeprazole and esomeprazole appear to be most likely to reduce the antiplatelet activity of clopidogrel and the FDA specifically warns against their concomitant use, it would be prudent to choose another PPI in patients taking clopidogrel.[17]

Pregnancy – PPIs are generally considered safe for use during pregnancy, but clinical data are limited. In a meta-analysis of 7 observational

Usual Adult Dosage[1]	Cost[2]
20-40 mg PO once/day	$333.40
	3306.80
	16.10[11]
20-40 mg PO once/day	3.30
	498.30
10-20 mg PO once/day	8.00
	524.70
	603.20
200 mcg PO bid, tid, or qid	82.50
	345.80
1 g PO qid[19]	36.00
	539.60

15. Contents of capsule should be sprinkled on soft food or liquid and consumed within 15 minutes.
16. FDA-approved only for prevention of NSAID-induced gastric ulcers.
17. Also available in combination with diclofenac (*Arthrotec*, and generics).
18. FDA-approved only for short-term treatment and maintenance therapy of duodenal ulcers.
19. Should be taken on an empty stomach.

studies, first-trimester PPI use (predominantly omeprazole) was not associated with an increased risk of congenital malformations.[18] A cohort study produced similar findings.[19]

ALGINATE — A polysaccharide derived from brown algae, alginate forms a floating foam/gel that acts as a physical barrier between gastric contents and the lower esophagus. In one randomized, placebo-controlled trial, addition of an alginate-based product (*Gaviscon Advance*; not available in the US) improved symptoms in patients who had heartburn or regurgitation despite standard-dose PPI treatment.[20] In the US, *Gaviscon* products contain aluminum hydroxide and magnesium carbonate; sodium alginate is listed as an inactive ingredient. *Gaviscon Advance* and other products available outside the US contain larger amounts of alginate.

ANTIREFLUX SURGERY — In patients with PPI-refractory and reflux-related chronic heartburn, antireflux surgery is an effective alternative to long-term pharmacologic treatment.[21]

PEPTIC ULCER DISEASE

Peptic ulcer disease (PUD) is most commonly caused by *Helicobacter pylori* infection. Use of nonsteroidal anti-inflammatory drugs (NSAIDs), including aspirin, is another common cause, especially in the US and other developed countries. Eradication of *H. pylori* can promote ulcer healing and prevent recurrence of gastric and duodenal ulcers.[22] It may also reduce the risk of gastric cancer in those who have a family history of the disease.[23]

PPI Treatment — All patients with PUD should be treated with a PPI for ulcer healing. If the underlying cause of PUD is identified and addressed (stopping the NSAID or eradicating *H. pylori*), long-term PPI treatment may not be needed. Long-term PPI treatment is recommended for patients with NSAID-induced PUD who are unable to stop taking NSAIDs (fixed-dose NSAID/PPI combinations are available for such patients) and for those whose PUD is not caused by *H. pylori* or NSAIDs.[12]

DIAGNOSIS OF *H. pylori* — Many diagnostic tests are available to identify *H. pylori* infection.[24, 25]

Urea Breath Tests – A urea breath test can be used for office-based diagnosis of active infection and confirmation of eradication. These tests typically have >90% sensitivity and specificity, and results are available within 10-20 minutes, but they require use of a mass spectrophotometer.

Stool Antigen Tests – Stool antigen enzyme immunoassay (EIA) testing also has >90% sensitivity and specificity and can test for active infection and eradication. It does not require special equipment and may be less expensive than urea breath tests. Stool samples can be used for molecular testing to determine antimicrobial susceptibility.

Serology – Serologic antibody tests for *H. pylori* lack sensitivity and specificity and do not differentiate between active and past infection. They cannot be used to confirm *H. pylori* eradication.

Endoscopy with Biopsy – *H. pylori* can be diagnosed from endoscopic biopsies using urease testing, histopathology, or culture. Urease testing of biopsy specimens has >90% sensitivity and specificity. Rapid tests are available that provide results in one hour. Histologic diagnosis from biopsy specimens has >95% sensitivity and specificity, but it takes longer and is more expensive than urease testing. Culture permits testing for antimicrobial susceptibility.

Drug Interference – The sensitivity of urea breath tests, stool antigen tests, and urease testing of biopsy specimens for *H. pylori* is reduced by use of PPIs, bismuth-containing products, and antibiotics. Patients should not take a PPI for at least 1-2 weeks or a bismuth-containing product or antibiotics for at least 4 weeks before these tests.

ERADICATION OF *H. pylori* — Preferred regimens for eradication of *H. pylori* infection are listed in Table 3.

In clinical trials, combinations of antibacterial drugs have been successful in eradicating *H. pylori*, but in clinical practice, eradication rates have been lower because of bacterial resistance and poor patient adherence to multi-drug regimens. Local resistance patterns and antimicrobial susceptibility testing should guide the selection of antibacterial drugs, but they are not readily available in the US.

Bismuth quadruple therapy (bismuth, metronidazole, tetracycline, and a PPI) is recommended for first-line treatment of *H. pylori* infection.[26] *H. pylori* resistance to tetracycline is rare, and adequate dosing of metronidazole can be effective even in the presence of *in vitro* resistance.[27]

Table 3. Preferred Regimens for *Helicobacter pylori* Infection[1]

Drug	Usual Adult Dosage[2]
Empiric Treatment	
Bismuth Quadruple Therapy[4]	
Bismuth subsalicylate[5]	262 or 525 mg PO qid
+ metronidazole	500 mg PO qid
+ tetracycline[7]	500 mg PO bid or qid
+ a PPI	See footnote 8
Rifabutin Triple Therapy[9]	
Rifabutin	150 mg bid
+ amoxicillin	1 g tid
+ esomeprazole or rabeprazole	40 mg bid
Susceptibility-Based Treatment	
Clarithromycin Triple Therapy	
Clarithromycin[10]	500 mg PO bid
+ amoxicillin	1 g PO bid
+ a PPI	See footnote 8
Clarithromycin[10]	500 mg PO bid
+amoxicillin	1 g PO bid
+vonoprazan[12]	20 mg PO bid
Levofloxacin Triple Therapy	
Levofloxacin	500 mg PO once/day
+ amoxicillin	1 g PO bid
+ a PPI	See footnote 8
Metronidazole Triple Therapy	
Metronidazole	500 mg PO bid
+ amoxicillin	1 g PO bid
+ a PPI	see footnote 8

PPI = proton pump inhibitor
1. Adapted from Y-C Lee et al. Annu Rev Med 2022; 73:183.
2. The optimal duration of treatment is 14 days.
3. Approximate WAC for the regimen based on 14 days' treatment with the generic products at the lowest usual adult dosage. PPI cost is for 28 tablets of *Prilosec OTC*. WAC = wholesaler acquisition cost or manufacturer's published price to wholesalers; WAC represents a published catalogue or list price and may not represent an actual transactional price. Source: AnalySource® Monthly. March 5, 2022. Reprinted with permission by First Databank, Inc. All rights reserved. ©2022. www.fdbhealth.com/policies/drug-pricing-policy.
4. The fixed-dose combination of bismuth subcitrate 140 mg, metronidazole 125 mg, and tetracycline 125 mg *(Pylera)* can be used, but it is only packaged as a 10-day supply; dosage is 3 capsules qid. A 10-day supply costs $921.50.
5. Or bismuth subcitrate 120-300 mg.

Comments	Cost[3]
▸ Preferred first-line option	$151.80[6]
▸ Alternative first-line option ▸ Can be used in treatment-naive patients or for salvage treatment	382.80
	138.60
▸ Should only be used in patients who reside in areas where clarithromycin resistance is <15% and in patients with no prior macrolide exposure for any indication[11] ▸ Clarithromycin triple therapy with vonoprazan was noninferior to triple therapy containing lansoprazole in patients with *H. pylori* susceptible to clarithromycin and amoxicillin	
▸ Levofloxacin resistance is a concern	53.20
▸ Metronidazole resistance is a concern	67.50

6. Cost for 14 days' treatment if generic tetracycline is used.
7. Generic tetracycline may not be available.
8. Esomeprazole 20 mg bid, lansoprazole 45 mg bid, omeprazole 40 mg bid, pantoprazole 40 mg bid, or rabeprazole 20 mg bid.
9. A fixed-dose combination of rifabutin 12.5 mg, omeprazole 10 mg, and amoxicillin 250 mg *(Talicia)* is available; dosage is 4 capsules tid. A 14-day supply costs $708.80.
10. Clarithromycin may increase the risk of cardiac adverse effects and death in patients with coronary artery disease (FDA Drug Safety Communication, February 2018).
11. Clarithromycin resistance rates are considered to be ≥15% unless local resistance patterns that show otherwise are available.
12. Vonoprazan is only available copackaged with amoxicillin *(Voquezna Dual Pak)* and with clarithromycin and amoxicillin *(Voquezna Triple Pak)* for treatment of *H. pylori*. Approximate WAC for a 14-day course of treatment is $812.00

Rifabutin triple therapy (rifabutin, amoxicillin, and a PPI) is an alternative option for empiric treatment of *H. pylori* infection. A fixed-dose combination of omeprazole, amoxicillin, and rifabutin *(Talicia)* eradicated *H. pylori* in about 80% of treatment-naive patients in two small clinical trials and is FDA-approved for treatment of *H. pylori* infection in adults.[28] Rifabutin-based triple therapy has not been compared directly to other regimens for first-line treatment of *H. pylori* infection in adults. Rates of *H. pylori* resistance to rifabutin have been low; whether more widespread use as part of a first-line regimen would increase resistance rates remains to be determined.

The efficacy of **clarithromycin** against *H. pylori* has been diminished by increasing antimicrobial resistance. Regimens containing clarithromycin should be used for first-line treatment only when antimicrobial susceptibility tests have shown that *H. pylori* is susceptible to the drug or in patients who have no history of macrolide use for any indication and reside in areas where *H. pylori* resistance to clarithromycin is known to be <15%. Limited data are available on *H. pylori* resistance rates in the US; they should be assumed to be ≥15% unless local resistance patterns show otherwise.

Adequate acid suppression with a **PPI** is associated with higher *H. pylori* cure rates. A higher intragastric pH improves antibiotic stability and bioavailability, resulting in higher drug concentrations. It also promotes *H. pylori* replication, making it more susceptible to antibiotic treatment. The potency of PPIs in maintaining a higher gastric pH varies from drug to drug (see Table 1).[8]

PPIs should be given twice daily (30-60 minutes before breakfast and dinner) for treatment of *H. pylori* infection. Dexlansoprazole can be given without regard to meals. Some experts recommend using high PPI doses (e.g., omeprazole 40 mg bid) for *H. pylori* eradication, especially in patients who are CYP2C19 ultra-rapid metabolizers.[29]

TREATMENT FAILURE — Testing for eradication of *H. pylori* should be performed at least 4 weeks after completion of therapy. Patients who are still infected should be treated with a different regimen. Bismuth quadruple therapy can be used in patients who initially received a regimen containing clarithromycin. Those who were initially treated with bismuth quadruple therapy can receive rifabutin triple therapy.

OTHER DRUGS — **Sucralfate**, an aluminum hydroxide complex of sucrose thought to act locally to protect ulcers from exposure to pepsin and gastric acid, has been used to heal peptic ulcers and as maintenance treatment to prevent recurrence. It may not be effective in relieving ulcer pain, must be taken multiple times per day, and can reduce the absorption of drugs taken concomitantly.

Misoprostol, a prostaglandin E1 analog, can prevent and heal gastro-duodenal ulcers in patients taking NSAIDs chronically, but it requires multiple daily doses and is not well tolerated.

Vonoprazan, a potassium-competitive acid blocker, copackaged with amoxicillin *(Voquezna Dual Pak)* and with amoxicillin and clarithromycin *(Voquezna Triple Pak)* was approved on May 3, 2022 by the FDA for treatment of *H. pylori* infection in adults. Vonoprazan is more rapidly absorbed, achieves a higher intragastric pH, and has a longer half-life (~7 hours vs ~1-2 hours) than conventional PPIs.[30] In one clinical trial, both vonoprazan dual therapy and triple therapy were noninferior to lansoprazole triple therapy (lansoprazole, amoxicillin, and clarithromycin) for eradication of *H. pylori* that was not resistant to clarithromycin or amoxicillin. In patients infected with clarithromycin-resistant strains, eradication rates were significantly higher with both vonoprazan regimens than with lansoprazole triple therapy but were relatively low with all 3 regimens.[31]

ADVERSE EFFECTS — The most common adverse effects associated with use of antibacterial drugs for treatment of *H. pylori* are diarrhea, nausea, vomiting, anorexia, and abdominal pain.

Bismuth subsalicylate can temporarily turn the tongue and stool black and can cause tinnitus. **Metronidazole** frequently causes a metallic taste and might cause a disulfiram-like reaction to alcohol; neurologic adverse effects, including seizures and neuropathy, have also been reported, particularly at high doses. **Tetracyclines** can cause GI adverse effects, vaginal candidiasis, photosensitivity, intracranial hypertension, and hyperpigmentation. Use of tetracyclines during tooth development (second and third trimesters of pregnancy, children ≤8 years old) can result in permanent discoloration of teeth. Because of their adverse effects on tooth and bone development, tetracyclines should not be used during pregnancy or in children ≤8 years old. **Levofloxacin** can cause severe hypoglycemia, delirium, agitation, nervousness, and disturbances in attention, memory, and orientation. It can also cause persistent or permanent peripheral neuropathy and an increased risk of pseudotumor cerebri syndrome. Tendinitis, tendon rupture, exacerbation of myasthenia gravis, *C. difficile* infection, and QT-interval prolongation and torsades de pointes can also occur. **Rifabutin** can cause brown-orange discoloration of urine, feces, saliva, sputum, perspiration, tears, and skin. It can rarely cause myelotoxicity (generally with higher-than-recommended doses or prolonged use) and uveitis. Serious, sometimes fatal, hypersensitivity reactions and *C. difficile* infection has been reported with use of rifabutin. **Clarithromycin** commonly causes taste disturbances that some patients find intolerable, and it can cause QT-interval prolongation.[32] The labeling of clarithromycin contains a warning about an increased risk of cardiac adverse events and death in patients with coronary artery disease.[33]

Sucralfate is generally well tolerated, but patients often complain about its metallic taste. It can cause constipation and, particularly in patients with renal impairment, aluminum toxicity. Abdominal pain and dose-related diarrhea, which can be severe, are the most common adverse effects of **misoprostol**. Severe nausea, dyspepsia, and flatulence can also occur. See pages 90-91 for adverse effects of **PPIs**.

DRUG INTERACTIONS — **Metronidazole** is an inhibitor of CYP2C9 and may increase serum concentrations of drugs metabolized by this isozyme, including warfarin. Coadministration of products containing calcium, magnesium, or iron can decrease absorption of **tetracycline**

and **levofloxacin**; either should be taken 2 hours before or 6 hours after these products. **Rifabutin** is an inducer of CYP3A4, 2C8 and 2C9 and can reduce serum concentrations of drugs that are metabolized by these isozymes. **Clarithromycin** is a strong inhibitor of CYP3A4 and P-glycoprotein (P-gp) and may increase serum concentrations of drugs that are CYP3A4 or P-gp substrates.[7] Taking clarithromycin with other drugs that prolong the QT interval, especially those metabolized by CYP3A4, can increase the risk of QT-interval prolongation and torsades de pointes.[33] **Sucralfate** decreases the absorption of many other drugs, including fluoroquinolones, tetracyclines, and levothyroxine; administration should be separated by at least 2 hours. See pages 91 and 94 for drug interactions of **PPIs**.

PREGNANCY — **Bismuth subsalicylate** is converted to bismuth and salicylic acid in the GI tract. Bismuth is minimally absorbed. The FDA has required new warnings in the labels of NSAIDs, including aspirin, advising against their use during pregnancy beginning at 20 weeks' gestation because of a risk of fetal renal dysfunction that could lead to low amniotic fluid levels and neonatal renal impairment. NSAIDs can cause premature closure of the ductus arteriosus and persistent neonatal pulmonary hypertension when used after 30 weeks' gestation.[34] **Metronidazole** is generally considered safe for use during pregnancy. An association between metronidazole exposure *in utero* and development of cleft lip was observed in one case-control study, but this finding has not been replicated in numerous other observational studies and meta-analyses.[35] **Tetracyclines** can cause fetal harm and reversible inhibition of bone growth when taken during pregnancy. **Levofloxacin** also should generally be avoided during pregnancy if possible. Fluoroquinolones have caused arthropathy in animal studies, but observational data in pregnant women suggest that teratogenic effects are unlikely to occur at therapeutic doses. **Rifabutin** and **clarithromycin** are generally not recommended for use during pregnancy. **Sucralfate** is minimally absorbed and does not appear to be associated with adverse fetal outcomes. **Misoprostol** is an abortifacient and should not be used in women who are or could become pregnant. See pages 94-95 for pregnancy considerations with **PPIs.**

1. J Maret-Ouda et al. Gastroesophageal reflux disease: a review. JAMA 2020; 324:2536.
2. PO Katz et al. ACG clinical guideline for the diagnosis and management of gastroesophageal reflux disease. Am J Gastroenterol 2022; 117:27.
3. E Ness-Jensen et al. Lifestyle intervention in gastroesophageal reflux disease. Clin Gastroenterol Hepatol 2016; 14:175.
4. M Singh et al. Weight loss can lead to resolution of gastroesophageal reflux disease symptoms: a prospective intervention trial. Obesity (Silver Spring) 2013; 21:284.
5. E Ness-Jensen et al. Weight loss and reduction in gastroesophageal reflux. A prospective population-based cohort study: the HUNT study. Am J Gastroenterol 2013; 108:376.
6. C Body and JA Christie. Gastrointestinal disease in pregnancy: nausea, vomiting, hyperemesis gravidarum, gastroesophageal reflux disease, constipation, and diarrhea. Gastroenterol Clin North Am 2016; 45:267.
7. Inhibitors and inducers of CYP enzymes, P-glycoprotein, and other transporters. Med Lett Drugs Ther 2021 October 20 (epub). Available at: http://secure.medicalletter.org/downloads/CYP_PGP_Tables.pdf.
8. DY Graham and A Tansel. Interchangeable use of proton pump inhibitors based on relative potency. Clin Gastroenterol Hepatol 2018; 16:800.
9. Safety of long-term PPI use. Med Lett Drugs Ther 2017; 59:131.
10. MF Vaezi et al. Complications of proton pump inhibitor therapy. Gastroenterology 2017; 153:35.
11. D Abrahami et al. Proton pump inhibitors and risk of gastric cancer: population-based cohort study. Gut 2022; 71:16.
12. DE Freedberg et al. The risks and benefits of long-term use of proton pump inhibitors: expert review and best practice advice from the American Gastroenterological Association. Gastroenterology 2017; 152:706.
13. T Furuta et al. Influence of CYP2C19 pharmacogenetic polymorphism on proton pump inhibitor-based therapies. Drug Metab Pharmacokinet 2005; 20:153.
14. RS Wedemeyer and H Blume. Pharmacokinetic drug interaction profiles of proton pump inhibitors: an update. Drug Saf 2014; 37:201.
15. SA Scott et al. Antiplatelet drug interactions with proton pump inhibitors. Expert Opin Drug Metab Toxicol 2014; 10:175.
16. SD Bouziana and K Tziomalos. Clinical relevance of clopidogrel-proton pump inhibitors interaction. World J Gastrointest Pharmacol Ther 2015; 6:17.
17. Drug interaction: clopidogrel and PPIs. Med Lett Drugs Ther 2017; 59:39.
18. SK Gill et al. The safety of proton pump inhibitors (PPIs) in pregnancy: a meta-analysis. Am J Gastroenterol 2009; 104:1541.
19. B Pasternak and A Hviid. Use of proton-pump inhibitors in early pregnancy and the risk of birth defects. N Engl J Med 2010; 363:2114.
20. C Reimer et al. Randomised clinical trial: alginate (Gaviscon Advance) vs. placebo as add-on therapy in reflux patients with inadequate response to a once daily proton pump inhibitor. Aliment Pharmacol Ther 2016; 43:899.
21. SJ Spechler et al. Randomized trial of medical versus surgical therapy for refractory heartburn. N Engl J Med 2019; 381:1513.
22. AC Ford et al. Eradication therapy for peptic ulcer disease in *Helicobacter pylori*-positive people. Cochrane Database Syst Rev 2016; 4:CD003840.

23. IJ Choi et al. Family history of gastric cancer and *Helicobacter pylori* treatment. N Engl J Med 2020; 382:427.
24. MP Dore et al. Dyspepsia: when and how to test for *Helicobacter pylori* infection. Gastroenterol Res Pract 2016; 2016:8463614.
25. Y-C Lee et al. Diagnosis and treatment of *Helicobacter pylori* infection. Annu Rev Med 2022; 73:183.
26. WD Chey et al. ACG clinical guideline: treatment of *Helicobacter pylori* infection. Am J Gastroenterol 2017; 112:212.
27. SC Shah et al. AGA clinical practice update on the management of refractory *Helicobacter pylori* infection: expert review. Gastroenterology 2021; 160:1831.
28. Talicia – a 3-drug combination for *Helicobacter pylori* infection. Med Lett Drugs Ther 2020; 62:83.
29. P Malfertheiner et al. Management of *Helicobacter pylori* infection–the Maastricht V/Florence consensus report. Gut 2017; 66:6.
30. DY Graham and MP Dore. Update on the use of vonoprazan: a competitive acid blocker. Gastroenterology 2018; 154:462.
31. WD Chey et al. Vonoprazan triple and dual therapy for *Helicobacter pylori* infection in the United States and Europe: randomized clinical trial. Gastroenterology 2022; 163:608.
32. RL Woosley et al. QT drugs list. Available at: www.crediblemeds.org. Accessed March 17, 2022.
33. FDA Drug Safety Communication: FDA review finds additional data supports the potential for increased long-term risks with antibiotic clarithromycin (Biaxin) in patients with heart disease. February 22, 2018. Available at: https://bit.ly/35m8rBk. Accessed March 17, 2022.
34. In brief: New warnings on NSAID use in pregnancy. Med Lett Drugs Ther 2020; 62:175.
35. O Sheehy et al. The use of metronidazole during pregnancy: a review of evidence. Curr Drug Saf 2015; 10:170.

| Lipid-Lowering Drugs

Original publication date − September 2022

Cholesterol management guidelines from the American College of Cardiology/American Heart Association Task Force were last published in 2019.[1]

STATINS — HMG-CoA reductase inhibitors (statins) remain the drugs of choice for most patients who require lipid-lowering therapy. Statins block the rate-limiting step in cholesterol synthesis. The subsequent reduction in hepatic cholesterol results in upregulation of low-density lipoprotein (LDL) receptor synthesis, increasing uptake and clearance of LDL-cholesterol (LDL-C) from the circulation.

Primary Prevention − Taken as an adjunct to diet, exercise, and smoking cessation, statins can reduce the risk of first cardiovascular events and death in patients at risk for atherosclerotic cardiovascular disease (ASCVD).[2]

Secondary Prevention − In a retrospective cohort study of ~500,000 patients with ASCVD, high-intensity statin therapy (rosuvastatin 20-40 mg, atorvastatin 40-80 mg) was associated with a survival advantage over lower-intensity statin therapy.[3]

Adverse Effects − All statins are generally well tolerated.[4] Patients who cannot tolerate one statin may tolerate another.

Key Points: Lipid-Lowering Drugs

▸ Statins are the lipid-lowering drugs of choice in most patients for treatment of hyperlipidemia and for prevention of cardiovascular disease.

▸ Statins can reduce the risk of a first cardiovascular event and death in patients at increased risk for atherosclerotic cardiovascular disease (ASCVD).

▸ Statins can decrease the risk of major coronary events and death in patients with ASCVD.

▸ Addition of ezetimibe to a statin can reduce the risk of secondary cardiovascular events.

▸ Addition of a PCSK9 inhibitor such as alirocumab or evolocumab to a statin can reduce LDL-C levels much more than a statin alone and can also reduce the risk of secondary cardiovascular events.

In clinical practice, muscle pain and weakness with or without increased creatine kinase levels are often reported in patients taking statins, but in a meta-analysis of 19 large double-blind trials, only ~7% of muscle symptoms reported by statin users were found to be attributable to the drugs.[5] Creatine kinase levels should be measured if myalgia occurs. Rarely, rhabdomyolysis and myoglobinuria leading to renal failure can occur.

An increase in serum aminotransferase levels to >3 times the upper limit of normal (ULN) occurs in 1-2% of patients receiving high-intensity statin therapy, but statin-induced liver damage is rare.

Statins have been associated with small increases in the incidence of new-onset diabetes and cognitive adverse effects, but their cardiovascular and mortality benefits far outweigh these risks.[6,7]

Drug Interactions – Statin-induced myopathy can be precipitated by drug interactions. Simvastatin and lovastatin undergo extensive first-pass metabolism by CYP3A4; concurrent use of a strong CYP3A4 inhibitor can dramatically increase their serum concentrations. Atorvastatin undergoes less first-pass metabolism by CYP3A4, but rhabdomyolysis has occurred with concurrent use of CYP3A4 inhibitors.[8]

Transporter proteins such as organic anion transporter polypeptides (OATP), P-glycoprotein (P-gp), and breast cancer resistance protein (BCRP) may play a role in statin pharmacokinetics; caution is advised when using statins concomitantly with drugs that inhibit these transporters.[9] Concurrent administration of cyclosporine increases serum concentrations of all statins and the risk of rhabdomyolysis, presumably through inhibition of CYP3A4, OATP, and P-gp. Concurrent use of gemfibrozil can increase statin concentrations and the risk of rhabdomyolysis, possibly through inhibition of OATP, and is not recommended.

Use of statins with high doses of niacin has been associated with myopathy and rhabdomyolysis; coadministration of simvastatin and lipid-modifying doses of niacin is not recommended in patients of Chinese descent, who are at increased risk for muscular adverse effects.[10]

In patients taking dabigatran etexilate (*Pradaxa*, and generics), concurrent use of simvastatin or lovastatin may increase the risk of major hemorrhage; the mechanism for this interaction is unclear.[11]

Bile acid sequestrants can interfere with the absorption of statins; they should be taken several hours before or after a statin. Colesevelam does not appear to interfere with the absorption of most statins.

Pregnancy and Lactation – Statins are no longer contraindicated for use during pregnancy. Multiple observational studies have not found an association between statin exposure *in utero* and major birth defects when controlling for other risks such as diabetes. The FDA still recommends stopping statins during pregnancy in most cases, but states that the benefits of continuing treatment may outweigh the risks in some patients, such as those with ASCVD or homozygous familial hypercholesterolemia (HoFH). Patients taking statins should not breastfeed; exposure to statins may disrupt lipid metabolism in the breastfed infant.[12]

Choice of a Statin – All FDA-approved statins reduce cardiovascular risk; the magnitude of the reduction increases with the magnitude of LDL-C lowering.[13] Atorvastatin and rosuvastatin at their highest approved doses are the most effective in lowering LDL-C levels. All statins except pitavastatin are available generically.[14,15] Dosage adjustments of atorvastatin and fluvastatin are not required in patients with severe renal impairment. Pravastatin, rosuvastatin, and pitavastatin are not metabolized by CYP isozymes to a clinically significant extent and are less likely to interact with other drugs.

CHOLESTEROL ABSORPTION INHIBITOR — Ezetimibe blocks transport and absorption of dietary and biliary cholesterol at the brush border of the small intestine. It reduces LDL-C levels by about 20-25%.

Efficacy – In a large, long-term (median follow-up of 6 years) secondary prevention trial (IMPROVE-IT), addition of ezetimibe 10 mg/day to simvastatin 40 mg/day resulted in a statistically significant reduction in cardiovascular events compared to addition of placebo in patients with recent acute coronary syndrome.[16] In a 3-year trial in 3780 patients with ASCVD, rosuvastatin 10 mg/day plus ezetimibe 10 mg/day was noninferior to monotherapy with rosuvastatin 20 mg/day in preventing cardiovascular death, major cardiovascular effects, or nonfatal stroke. The combination also lowered LDL-cholesterol significantly more and was less likely to be discontinued.[17]

Adverse Effects – Ezetimibe is generally well tolerated. Diarrhea, arthralgia, rhabdomyolysis, hepatitis, pancreatitis, and thrombocytopenia have been reported, but causal relationships are unclear. In IMPROVE-IT, the incidence of adverse events with ezetimibe plus a statin was similar to that with a statin alone.[16] Patients with moderate to severe hepatic impairment (Child-Pugh B or C) should not take ezetimibe.

Drug Interactions – Ezetimibe may increase the anticoagulant effect of warfarin. Concurrent use of ezetimibe and cyclosporine increases serum concentrations of both drugs. Concurrent use of gemfibrozil and ezetimibe can increase the risk of cholelithiasis and is contraindicated.

Bile acid sequestrants interfere with ezetimibe absorption; they should be taken several hours before or after taking ezetimibe.

Pregnancy and Lactation – Skeletal anomalies were observed in the offspring of rats and rabbits given 10-150 times the usual human dose of ezetimibe. The drug has been detected in the milk of lactating rats. No data are available on the presence of ezetimibe in human breast milk or its effects on the breastfed infant or milk production.

PCSK9 INHIBITORS — Proprotein convertase subtilisin/kexin type 9 (PCSK9) binds to LDL receptors on hepatocytes, promoting receptor degradation, preventing LDL-C clearance from the circulation, and increasing serum concentrations of LDL-C. Alirocumab and evolocumab are subcutaneously injected monoclonal antibodies that bind to PCSK9 and prevent it from binding to LDL receptors, increasing receptor density and clearance of circulating LDL-C.[18,19]

Efficacy – Adding alirocumab or evolocumab to a statin reduces LDL-C levels by 50-60%.[20,21] A meta-analysis of 24 trials found that addition of alirocumab or evolocumab to standard lipid-lowering therapy in high-risk patients decreased the risk of adverse cardiovascular events over a follow-up period of 6-36 months.[22] Both alirocumab and evolocumab have been associated with a reduction in atherosclerosis when given after a myocardial infarction.[23,24]

Adverse Effects – Both alirocumab and evolocumab appear to be well tolerated. Myalgia, rash, urticaria, and mild injection-site reactions have been reported. Treatment with a PCSK9 inhibitor can result in very low LDL-C levels (<25 mg/dL), but no associated adverse events have been reported. Neither drug was associated with cognitive adverse events in placebo-controlled trials.[10,25,26]

Pregnancy and Lactation – A few studies have suggested a possible association between PCSK9 inhibition during pregnancy and fetal neural tube defects.[27,28] Whether alirocumab or evolocumab is present in human breast milk is not known, but human IgG antibodies generally cross the placenta and can be found in breast milk.

PCSK9-DIRECTED SMALL INTERFERING RNA — Inclisiran is a subcutaneously injected chemically modified, double-stranded, small interfering RNA that directs catalytic breakdown of mRNA for PCSK9, preventing PCSK9 synthesis and degradation of LDL-C receptors.[29]

Efficacy – In clinical trials in adults with ASCVD or heterozygous familial hypercholesterolemia (HeFH), inclisiran reduced LDL-C levels by about 50% when added to maximally tolerated statin therapy.[30,31] Its effects on clinical outcomes remain to be determined.[32]

Adverse Effects – The most common adverse effects of inclisiran in clinical trials were injection-site reactions, arthralgia, urinary tract infections, diarrhea, bronchitis, extremity pain, and dyspnea.

Pregnancy and Lactation – No data are available on use of inclisiran during pregnancy or breastfeeding. A few studies have suggested a possible association between PCSK9 inhibition during pregnancy and fetal neural tube defects.[27,28]

FISH OILS — Long-chain omega-3 polyunsaturated fatty acids (PUFAs) can reduce elevated fasting triglyceride concentrations by 20-50% by decreasing hepatic triglyceride production and increasing triglyceride clearance.[33] Long-term use may increase HDL-C levels.

Efficacy – Most clinical trials of fish oil supplements have not provided any convincing evidence that they prevent cardiovascular disease or improve outcomes in patients who already have it.[34,35]

A combination of the omega-3 PUFAs eicosapentaenoic acid and docosahexaenoic acid (EPA/DHA), available by prescription, is FDA-approved for treatment of severe hypertriglyceridemia. Daily doses of 3-12 g can lower triglycerides by 20-50%. The combination has not been shown to prevent pancreatitis, which is a major concern in patients with very high triglycerides.

Icosapent ethyl, another prescription omega-3 PUFA product, is also FDA-approved for treatment of severe hypertriglyceridemia. In a randomized double-blind trial in patients with hypertriglyceridemia and diabetes or ASCVD (REDUCE-IT), triglyceride levels were reduced and the incidence of cardiovascular events was decreased significantly with icosapent ethyl compared to placebo. The validity of this trial is uncertain because the results of a biomarker substudy suggested that the mineral oil placebo could have increased the incidence of cardio-vascular events.[36-38] Whether icosapent ethyl can prevent pancreatitis remains to be determined.

Adverse Effects – Adverse effects of fish oils have included eructation, dyspepsia, and an unpleasant aftertaste. Worsening glycemic control has been reported in patients with diabetes taking high doses. Inhibition of platelet aggregation and increased bleeding time can occur with high doses of fish oils; whether they can cause clinically significant bleeding is unclear. In REDUCE-IT, bleeding and atrial fibrillation occurred more often with icosapent ethyl than with placebo.[39]

Drug Interactions – Use of fish oils concomitantly with anticoagulant or antiplatelet drugs can increase the risk of bleeding.

Pregnancy and Lactation – Omega-3 PUFAs given at 7 times the recommended human dose were embryocidal in rats. Omega-3 PUFAs are secreted into human breast milk.

BILE ACID SEQUESTRANTS — The resins cholestyramine and colestipol and the hydrophilic polymer colesevelam hydrochloride prevent reabsorption of bile acids, resulting in increased conversion of cholesterol to bile acids, depletion of intrahepatic cholesterol, and upregulation of LDL receptor synthesis. These drugs can lower LDL-C levels by up to 20% and increase HDL-C levels.

Table 1. Some Lipid-Lowering Drugs

Drug	Some Formulations
Statins	
Atorvastatin – generic	10, 20, 40, 80 mg tabs
Lipitor (Pfizer)	
Fluvastatin – generic	20, 40 mg caps
extended-release – generic	80 mg ER tabs
Lescol XL (Novartis)	
Lovastatin – generic	10, 20, 40 mg tabs
extended-release – *Altoprev* (Covis)	20, 40, 60 mg ER tabs
Pitavastatin calcium[6] –	1, 2, 4 mg tabs
Livalo (Kowa)	
Pitavastatin magnesium[6] –	1, 2, 4 mg tabs
Zypitamag (Medicure)	
Pravastatin – generic	10, 20, 40, 80 mg tabs
Rosuvastatin – generic	5, 10, 20, 40 mg tabs
Crestor (AstraZeneca)	
Ezallor Sprinkle (Sun)	5, 10, 20, 40 mg sprinkle caps
Simvastatin – generic	5, 10, 20, 40, 80 mg tabs
Zocor (Merck)	10, 20, 40 mg tabs
Flolipid (Salerno)	20 mg/5 mL, 40 mg/5 mL susp

ER = extended-release; susp = suspension

1. FDA-approved dosage. Some expert clinicians use lower doses for initial treatment of patients with only modest elevations of LDL-C or a history of poor tolerance to these drugs. For patients who require a large reduction in LDL-C, some would use higher doses initially. Statins are generally most effective when taken in the evening. Dosage adjustments may be needed for patients with renal or hepatic impairment.
2. The listed ranges correspond to the initial and maximum dosages. Statin regimens that lower LDL-C ≥50% are considered high-intensity therapy. Those that lower LDL-C 30-49% are considered moderate-intensity therapy, and those that lower LDL-C <30% are considered low-intensity therapy. LDL-C reductions may vary significantly among individuals.
3. Approximate WAC for 30 days' treatment with the lowest usual initial adult dosage. WAC = wholesaler acquisition cost or manufacturer's published price to wholesalers; WAC represents a published catalogue or list price and may not represent an actual transactional price. Source: AnalySource® Monthly. August 5, 2022. Reprinted with permission by First Databank, Inc. All rights reserved. ©2022. www.fdbhealth.com/policies/drug-pricing-policy.

Usual Adult Dosage[1]	Average LDL-C Reduction[2]	Cost[3]
Initial: 10-20 mg PO once/day	35-40%	$5.10
Maximum: 80 mg PO once/day	50-60%	346.00
Initial: 40 mg PO bid	30-35%	260.50
Maximum: 40 mg PO bid	30-35%	
Initial: 80 mg PO once/day	35-40%	173.40
Maximum: 80 mg PO once/day	35-40%	339.10
Initial: 20 mg PO once/day	25-30%	13.90
Maximum: 80 mg PO once/day[4,5]	35-40%	
Initial: 20 mg PO once/day	20-25%	1083.10
Maximum: 60 mg PO once/day[5]	40-45%	
Initial: 2 mg PO once/day[7]	35-40%	
Maximum: 4 mg PO once/day[7]	40-45%	319.70
Initial: 2 mg PO once/day[7]	35-40%	
Maximum: 4 mg PO once/day[7]	40-45%	232.50
Initial: 40 mg PO once/day[8]	30-35%	11.50
Maximum: 80 mg PO once/day	35-40%	
Initial: 10-20 mg PO once/day[9,10]	45-50%	9.90
Maximum: 40 mg PO once/day[10,11]	50-60%	276.50
		99.20
Initial: 10-20 mg PO once/day[12,13]	35-40%	3.00
Maximum: 40 mg PO once/day[13]	45-50%	145.40
		121.70

4. Or 40 mg bid.
5. Use doses >20 mg/day cautiously in patients with severe renal impairment.
6. *Livalo* and *Zypitamag* are considered bioequivalent.
7. 1 mg/day initially, 2 mg/day maximum in patients with moderate or severe renal impairment.
8. 10 mg initially for patients with severe renal impairment.
9. Higher serum concentrations of rosuvastatin have been reported in Asian patients, especially those of East Asian descent (BK Birmingham et al; Eur J Clin Pharmacol 2015; 71:329); an initial rosuvastatin dose of 5 mg is recommended.
10. Patients with severe renal impairment not on hemodialysis should start with 5 mg/day of rosuvastatin and not exceed 10 mg/day.
11. Maximum rosuvastatin dose is 20 mg/day in Asian patients (E Lee et al. Clin Pharmacol 2005; 78:330).
12. Patients with severe renal impairment should start with 5 mg.
13. The maximum dose of simvastatin is 10 mg if taken with diltiazem, dronedarone, or verapamil and 20 mg if taken with amiodarone, amlodipine, or ranolazine.

Continued on next page

Table 1. Some Lipid-Lowering Drugs (continued)

Drug	Some Formulations
Cholesterol Absorption Inhibitor	
Ezetimibe – generic	10 mg tabs
Zetia (Organon)	
Cholesterol Absorption Inhibitor/Statin Combinations	
Ezetimibe/rosuvastatin – generic	10/5, 10/10, 10/20, 10/40 mg tabs
Roszet (Althera)	
Ezetimibe/simvastatin – generic	10/10, 10/20, 10/40, 10/80 mg tabs
Vytorin (Organon)	
ACL Inhibitor	
Bempedoic acid – *Nexletol* (Esperion)	180 mg tabs
ACL Inhibitor/Cholesterol Absorption Inhibitor	
Bempedoic acid/ezetimibe –	
Nexlizet (Esperion)	180/10 mg tabs
PCSK9 Inhibitors	
Alirocumab – *Praluent* (Regeneron)	75, 150 mg/mL single-use pens
Evolocumab – *Repatha* (Amgen)	140 mg/mL single-use prefilled syringes
Repatha Sureclick	140 mg/mL single-use prefilled autoinjectors
Repatha Pushtronex	420 mg/3.5 mL single-use infusors with prefilled cartridges
PCSK9-Directed Small Interfering RNA (siRNA)	
Inclisiran – *Leqvio* (Novartis)	284 mg/1.5 mL single-use prefilled syringes

ACL = adenosine triphosphate-citrate lyase; PCSK9 = proprotein convertase subtilisin/kexin type 9
14. Not recommended for use in patients with moderate to severe hepatic impairment.
15. The 300-mg dose is given as 2 consecutive 150-mg injections at different sites.
16. Alone or when added to statin therapy.
17. Cost for dosage q4 weeks or once monthly.
18. Dosage for patients with heterozygous familial hypercholesterolemia (HeFH) or atherosclerotic cardiovascular disease (ASCVD). Dosage for patients with homozygous familial hypercholesterolemia (HoFH) is 420 mg SC once monthly.

Usual Adult Dosage[1]	Average LDL-C Reduction[2]	Cost[3]
10 mg PO once/day	20-25%	$9.50
		361.90
Initial: 10/10-10/20 mg PO once/day[9,10]	55-60%	35.00
Maximum: 10/40 mg PO once/day[10,11]	60-70%	35.00
Initial: 10/10-10/20 mg PO once/day[13]	40-50%	69.40
Maximum: 10/40 mg PO once/day[13]	50-60%	358.40
180 mg PO once/day	15-20%	384.40
180/10 mg PO once/day[14]	35-40%	384.40
Initial: 75 mg SC q2 wks or 300 mg SC q4 wks[15]	45-50%[16]	477.40[17]
Maximum: 150 mg SC q2 wks or 300 mg SC q4 wks[15]	50-60%[16]	
Initial: 140 mg SC q2 wks or 420 mg SC once/month[18,19]	55-60%[16]	779.70[17]
Maximum: 420 mg SC once/month[19]		779.70[17]
		563.10[17]
284 mg SC at months 0 and 3, then q6 months[20]	40-50%	6500.00[21]

19. The 420-mg dose is given as a single dose through the infusor or as three consecutive 140-mg injections within 30 minutes.
20. Must be administered by a healthcare provider.
21. Cost for 2 doses per year; the cost for the first year of treatment (3 doses) is $9750.

Continued on next page

Table 1. Some Lipid-Lowering Drugs (continued)

Drug	Some Formulations
Bile Acid Sequestrants	
Cholestyramine – generic	4 g packets; 4 g/scoop
Questran (Par)	
Cholestyramine light[22] – generic	4 g packets; 4 g/scoop
Prevalite (Upsher-Smith)	
Colesevelam – generic	625 mg tabs; 3.75 g packets
Welchol (Daiichi Sankyo)	
Colestipol – generic	1 g tabs; 5 g packets; 5 g/scoop
Colestid (Pfizer)	1 g tabs; 5, 7.5 g packets; 5 g/scoop
Fibric Acid Derivatives	
Fenofibrate – generic	54, 160 mg tabs
Fenoglide[27] (Santarus)	40, 120 mg tabs
Lipofen[27] (Kowa)	50, 150 mg caps
micronized[26] – generic	43, 67, 134, 200 mg caps
Antara[27] (Lupin)	30, 90 mg caps
nanocrystallized[28] – generic	48, 145 mg tabs
Tricor (AbbVie)	
Fenofibric acid – generic	35, 105 mg tabs
delayed-release – generic	45, 135 mg delayed-release caps
Trilipix (AbbVie)	
Gemfibrozil – generic	600 mg tabs
Lopid (Pfizer)	
Niacin	
Niacin immediate-release – generic[30]	500 mg caps; 500 mg tabs
Niacor (Avondale)	500 mg tabs
extended-release – generic	500, 750, 1000 mg ER tabs
Niaspan (AbbVie)	
sustained-release – *Slo-Niacin*	250, 500, 750 mg SR tabs
(Main Pointe)[30]	

ER = extended-release
22. Contains aspartame instead of sucrose.
23. Cost of a 30-day supply of packets.
24. Should be taken with food.
25. Dosage for granules.
26. Dosage for tablets.

Usual Adult Dosage[1]	Average LDL-C Reduction[2]	Cost[3]
8 g PO once/day or 4 g PO bid	15-20%	$109.80[23]
		341.20[23]
		106.20[23]
		123.00[23]
3.75 g PO once/day or 1.875 g PO bid[24]	15-20%	418.00[23]
		735.90[23]
10 g PO once/day or 5 g PO bid[25] or 2-16 g PO once/day or divided[26]	15-20%	158.60[23]
		421.20[23]
160 mg PO once/day[24]	5-10%[29]	35.30
120 mg PO once/day[24]		1113.20
150 mg PO once/day[24]		284.50
200 mg PO once/day[24]		24.00
90 mg PO once/day		507.90
145 mg PO once/day		42.50
		31.00
105 mg PO once/day	5-10%[29]	72.10
135 mg PO once/day		39.80
		270.70
600 mg PO bid	5-10%[29]	12.30
		77.40
1000 mg PO tid	5-25%	4.10
1000-2000 mg PO bid or tid		745.20
1000-2000 mg PO once/day[31]		65.80
		274.20
750 mg PO once/day		14.50

27. Also available generically.
28. Nanocrystallized and micronized formulations may result in greater solubility and improved bioavailability compared to nonmicronized formulations.
29. LDL-C levels may increase when triglyceride levels are decreased.
30. Available over the counter.
31. Should be taken with a low-fat snack at bedtime.

Continued on next page

Table 1. Some Lipid-Lowering Drugs (continued)	
Drug	**Some Formulations**
Fish Oils	
Icosapent ethyl – generic	1 g caps[32]
Vascepa (Amarin)	500 mg, 1 g caps[32]
Omega-3 acid ethyl esters – generic	1 g caps[34]
Lovaza (GSK)	

32. EPA content.
33. FDA-approved dosage for treating hypertriglyceridemia (≥500 mg/dL).

Efficacy – In a double-blind trial in 3806 men 35-59 years old with primary hypercholesterolemia, cholestyramine monotherapy for an average of 7.4 years significantly decreased the incidence of coronary death or nonfatal myocardial infarction compared to placebo.[32]

Adverse Effects – Constipation occurs frequently with colestipol and cholestyramine and may be accompanied by heartburn, nausea, eructation, and bloating. Colesevelam is better tolerated.

Bile acid sequestrants may further increase plasma triglyceride levels in patients with hypertriglyceridemia; they should generally be avoided in patients with triglyceride levels >300 mg/dL. Colesevelam is contraindicated for use in those with triglyceride levels >500 mg/dL.

Drug Interactions – Bile acid sequestrants can interfere with the absorption of other oral drugs, including statins and ezetimibe; they should be taken several hours apart. Colesevelam does not appear to interfere with the absorption of most statins. Bile acid sequestrants can also interfere with the absorption of fat-soluble vitamins.

Pregnancy and Lactation – Bile acid sequestrants may interfere with maternal absorption of vitamins. Cholestyramine, colestipol, and

Usual Adult Dosage[1]	Average LDL-C Reduction[2]	Cost[3]
2 g PO bid[24,33]	0-5%[29]	$298.40 354.60
4 g PO once/day or 2 g PO bid[33]	See footnote 29	132.40 669.20

34. Each 1000-mg capsule contains about 465 mg EPA and about 375 mg DHA (total 900 mg polyunsaturated fatty acids [PUFAs]).

colesevelam are not absorbed systemically and are not expected to be present in human breast milk.

ACL INHIBITOR—The oral adenosine triphosphate-citrate lyase (ACL) inhibitor bempedoic acid is FDA-approved for use alone and in a fixed-dose combination with ezetimibe as an adjunct to maximally tolerated statin therapy in adults with heterozygous familial hypercholesterolemia (HeFH) or established ASCVD who require additional lowering of LDL-C. Bempedoic acid inhibits ACL, an enzyme involved in hepatic cholesterol synthesis. The reduction in LDL-C causes upregulation of LDL receptors, increasing clearance of LDL-C from the circulation.[40]

Efficacy – In clinical trials in patients with HeFH, ASCVD, and/or multiple cardiovascular risk factors, addition of bempedoic acid to maximally tolerated statin therapy, with or without ezetimibe, resulted in further LDL-C reductions of ~15-20%.[41-43] The effects of the drug on clinical outcomes remain to be determined.[32]

Adverse Effects – Adverse effects of bempedoic acid in clinical trials included upper respiratory tract infection, muscle spasms, back pain, extremity pain, abdominal pain or discomfort, anemia, and elevated hepatic enzymes. The drug inhibits renal tubular organic anion transporter 2 (OAT2) and may increase serum uric acid levels and the risk of developing gout; treatment with urate-lowering drugs may be needed. Bempedoic acid has been associated with an increased risk of benign prostatic hyperplasia. Tendon rupture occurred in 0.5% of patients taking the drug.

Drug Interactions – Coadministration of bempedoic acid with simvastatin or pravastatin increases serum concentrations of the statin. Concomitant use with >20 mg/day of simvastatin or >40 mg/day of pravastatin may increase the risk of myopathy and is not recommended.

Pregnancy and Lactation – No data are available on the use of bempedoic acid in pregnant or breastfeeding women. Fetal skeletal variations, reduced fetal weight, and fetal loss have been reported in animal studies. The manufacturer recommends that women avoid breastfeeding while taking bempedoic acid.

FIBRIC ACID DERIVATIVES — Fibrates are primarily used to lower triglycerides. They activate the nuclear transcription factor peroxisome proliferator-activated receptor-alpha (PPARα), which regulates genes that control lipid and glucose metabolism, inflammation, and endothelial function. Gemfibrozil, fenofibrate, and fenofibric acid decrease triglyceride and VLDL-C levels, usually by 25-50%, and may increase HDL-C levels. They may decrease LDL-C levels in patients with low to normal triglycerides, but may increase LDL-C levels when used to treat hypertriglyceridemia.[44]

Efficacy – Gemfibrozil is the only fibrate with demonstrated beneficial effects on cardiovascular outcomes,[45] but its use with statins can increase the risk of myopathy and is not recommended. Fenofibrate may be more effective than gemfibrozil in lowering LDL-C and triglyceride levels, but there is no evidence that addition of fenofibrate to a statin improves cardiovascular outcomes.

Adverse Effects – GI adverse effects are common with fibrates. Cholelithiasis, hepatitis, and myositis can occur. A paradoxical severe decrease in HDL-C levels has been reported; if this occurs, the fibrate should be stopped. Fibrates are contraindicated in patients with liver or gallbladder disease. Fenofibrate can increase serum creatinine levels; the dose should be reduced in patients with mild to moderate renal impairment and the drug should not be used in those with severe renal impairment.

Drug Interactions – Fibrates may potentiate the effects of warfarin and antihyperglycemic drugs. Gemfibrozil can increase serum concentrations of statins, possibly through inhibition of OATP, increasing the risk of rhabdomyolysis; concurrent use is not recommended. Concurrent use of gemfibrozil and ezetimibe can increase the risk of cholelithiasis and is contraindicated.

Pregnancy and Lactation – Adverse effects on fetal development have been observed with gemfibrozil and fenofibrate in animal studies. No data are available on the presence of fibric acid derivatives in human breast milk or their effects on the breastfed infant or milk production.

NIACIN — Niacin (nicotinic acid) has favorable effects on all plasma lipoproteins and lipids. It also decreases plasma levels of lipoprotein(a), a marker of cardiovascular risk.[46] There is no convincing evidence, however, that adding niacin to a statin improves cardiovascular outcomes.

Efficacy – In a trial in patients with ASCVD (HPS2-THRIVE), addition of niacin to statin therapy did not significantly reduce the incidence of first major vascular events.[47]

Adverse Effects – Niacin can cause flushing, pruritus, GI distress, blurred vision, fatigue, glucose intolerance, hyperuricemia, hepatic toxicity, exacerbation of peptic ulcers and, rarely, dry eyes or skin hyperpigmentation. Some adverse effects, particularly flushing, are more common with the immediate-release formulation.

Drug Interactions – Use of statins with high doses of niacin has been associated with myopathy and rhabdomyolysis; coadministration of simvastatin and lipid-modifying doses of niacin is not recommended in patients of Chinese descent, who are at increased risk for muscular adverse effects.[10]

Pregnancy and Lactation – Niacin can cross the placenta and is not recommended for use during pregnancy or while breastfeeding.

HoFH — Homozygous familial hypercholesterolemia (HoFH), a rare inherited condition (estimated prevalence 1:160,000 to 1:300,000) that is usually caused by defects in the LDL receptor gene, causes very high LDL-C levels, cutaneous xanthoma soon after birth, and, without treatment, premature cardiovascular disease and death in childhood.

The PCSK9 inhibitor **evolocumab** *(Repatha)* is FDA-approved for treatment of HoFH in patients ≥10 years old. In a randomized trial, it reduced LDL-C levels by 31% compared to placebo in patients with residual LDL-receptor activity.[48]

Lomitapide *(Juxtapid)*, an oral microsomal triglyceride transfer protein inhibitor, is FDA-approved for treatment of HoFH in adults. It can lower LDL-C by 40% in patients with HoFH already taking maximum doses of other lipid-lowering drugs.[49] Serious adverse effects, particularly hepatotoxicity, can occur.

Evinacumab *(Evkeeza)*, an angiopoietin-like 3 (ANGPTL3) inhibitor, is FDA-approved for treatment of HoFH in patients ≥12 years old. ANGPTL3 is a protein expressed primarily in the liver that inhibits lipoprotein lipase and endothelial lipase. Inhibition of ANGPTL3 decreases LDL-C, HDL-C, and triglyceride levels. In a double-blind trial, 65 patients with clinically or genetically diagnosed HoFH (mean baseline LDL-C 255 mg/dL) were randomized to receive IV infusions of evinacumab 15 mg/kg or placebo every 4 weeks; the change in LDL-C level from baseline to week 24, the primary endpoint, was -47.1% with evinacumab vs +1.9% with placebo.[50] In clinical trials, the most common adverse effects of evinacumab were nasopharyngitis, influenza-like illness, infusion reactions, dizziness, rhinorrhea, and nausea. Anaphylaxis occurred in one patient.[51]

1. SM Grundy et al. 2018 AHA/ACC/AACVPR/AAPA/ABC/ACPM/ADA/AGS/APhA/ASPC/NLA/PCNA guideline on the management of blood cholesterol: a report of the American College of Cardiology/American Heart Association Task Force on clinical practice guidelines. J Am Coll Cardiol 2019; 73:e285.
2. US Preventive Services Task Force. Statin use for the primary prevention of cardiovascular disease in adults. US Preventive Services Task Force recommendation statement. JAMA 2022; 328:746.
3. F Rodriguez et al. Association between intensity of statin therapy and mortality in patients with atherosclerotic cardiovascular disease. JAMA Cardiol 2017; 2:47.
4. CB Newman et al. Statin safety and associated adverse events: a scientific statement from the American Heart Association. Arterioscler Thromb Vasc Biol 2019; 39:e38.
5. Cholesterol Treatment Trialists' Collaboration. Effect of statin therapy on muscle symptoms: an individual participant meta-analysis of large-scale, randomised, double-blind trials. Lancet 2022 August 29 (epub).
6. JG Robinson. Statins and diabetes risk: how real is it and what are the mechanisms? Curr Opin Lipidol 2015; 26:228.
7. DB Rosoff et al. Mendelian randomization study of PCSK9 and HMG-CoA reductase inhibition and cognitive function. J Am Coll Cardiol 2022; 80:653.
8. Inhibitors and inducers of CYP enzymes, P-glycoprotein, and other transporters. Med Lett Drugs Ther 2021 October 20 (epub). Available at: medicalletter.org/downloads/CYP_PGP_Tables.pdf.
9. BS Wiggins et al. Recommendations for management of clinically significant drug-drug interactions with statins and select agents used in patients with cardiovascular disease: a scientific statement from the American Heart Association. Circulation 2016; 134:e468.
10. The AIM-HIGH Investigators. Niacin in patients with low HDL cholesterol levels receiving intensive statin therapy. N Engl J Med 2011; 365:2255.
11. Drug interaction: dabigatran (Pradaxa) and statins. Med Lett Drugs Ther 2017; 59:26.
12. FDA Drug Safety Communication. FDA requests removal of strongest warning against using cholesterol-lowering statins during pregnancy; still advises most pregnant patients should stop taking statins. August 30, 2021. Available at: https://bit.ly/3A6cvlN. Accessed August 31, 2022.
13. MG Silverman et al. Association between lowering LDL-C and cardiovascular risk reduction among different therapeutic interventions: a systematic review and meta-analysis. JAMA 2016; 316:1289.
14. Pitavastatin (Livalo) – the seventh statin. Med Lett Drugs Ther 2010; 52:57.
15. In brief: Pitavastatin magnesium (Zypitamag) for hyperlipidemia. Med Lett Drugs Ther 2018; 60:106.
16. CP Cannon et al. Ezetimibe added to statin therapy after acute coronary syndromes. N Engl J Med 2015; 372:2387.
17. B-K Kim et al. Long-term efficacy and safety of moderate-intensity statin with ezetimibe combination therapy versus high-intensity statin monotherapy in patients

with atherosclerotic cardiovascular disease (RACING): a randomized, open-label, non-inferiority trial. Lancet 2022; 400:380.

18. Alirocumab (Praluent) to lower LDL-cholesterol. Med Lett Drugs Ther 2015; 57:113.

19. Evolocumab (Repatha) – a second PCSK9 inhibitor to lower LDL-cholesterol. Med Lett Drugs Ther 2015; 57:140.

20. JG Robinson et al. Efficacy and safety of alirocumab in reducing lipids and cardiovascular events. N Engl J Med 2015; 372:1489.

21. MS Sabatine et al. Evolocumab and clinical outcomes in patients with cardiovascular disease. N Engl J Med 2017; 376:1713.

22. AF Schmidt et al. PCSK9 monoclonal antibodies for the primary and secondary prevention of cardiovascular disease. Cochrane Database Syst Rev 2020; 10:CD011748.

23. L Raber et al. Effect of alirocumab added to high-intensity statin therapy on coronary atherosclerosis in patients with acute myocardial infarction: the PACMAN-AMI randomized clinical trial. JAMA 2022; 327:1771.

24. SJ Nicholls et al. Effect of evolocumab on coronary plaque phenotype and burden in statin-treated patients following myocardial infarction. JACC Cardiovasc Imaging 2022; 15:1308.

25. RP Giugliano et al. Cognitive function in a randomized trial of evolocumab. N Engl J Med 2017; 377:633.

26. PD Harvey et al. No evidence of neurocognitive adverse events associated with alirocumab treatment in 3340 patients from 14 randomized phase 2 and 3 controlled trials: a meta-analysis of individual patient data. Eur Heart J 2018; 39:374.

27. Z Yuan. Dysregulated expressions of PCSK9 are associated with neural tube defects. Atherosclerosis Supplements 2018; 32:143.

28. RN Jerome et al. Using human 'experiments of nature' to predict drug safety issues: an example with PCSK9 inhibitors. Drug Saf 2018; 41:303.

29. Inclisiran (Leqvio) for LDL-cholesterol lowering. Med Lett Drugs Ther 2022; 64:43.

30. KK Ray et al. Two phase 3 trials of inclisiran in patients with elevated LDL cholesterol. N Engl J Med 2020; 382:1507.

31. FJ Raal et al. Inclisiran for the treatment of heterozygous familial hypercholesterolemia. N Engl J Med 2020; 382:1520.

32. DM Lloyd-Jones et al. 2022 ACC expert consensus decision pathway on the role of nonstatin therapies for LDL-cholesterol lowering in the management of atherosclerotic cardiovascular disease risk: a report of the American College of Cardiology Solution Set Oversight Committee. J Am Coll Cardiol 2022 August 25 (epub).

33. Fish oil supplements. Med Lett Drugs Ther 2012; 54:83.

34. Risk and Prevention Study Collaborative Group. n-3 fatty acids in patients with multiple cardiovascular risk factors. N Engl J Med 2013; 368:1800.

35. JE Manson et al. Marine n-3 fatty acids and prevention of cardiovascular disease and cancer. N Engl J Med 2019; 380:23.

36. DL Bhatt et al. Cardiovascular risk reduction with icosapent ethyl for hypertriglyceridemia. N Engl J Med 2019; 380:11.

37. PM Ridker et al. Effects of randomized treatment with icosapent ethyl and a mineral oil comparator on interleukin 1-β, interleukin-6, C-reactive protein, oxidized low-density

lipoprotein cholesterol, homocysteine, lipoprotein(a), and lipoprotein-associated phospholipase A2: a REDUCE-IT biomarker substudy. Circulation 2022; 146:372.

38. RA Harrington. Trials and tribulations of randomized clinical trials. Circulation 2022; 146:380.

39. B Gencer et al. Effects of long-term marine Ω-3 fatty acids supplementation on the risk of atrial fibrillation in randomized controlled trials of cardiovascular outcomes: a systematic review and meta-analysis. Circulation 2021; 144:1981.

40. Bempedoic acid (Nexletol) for lowering LDL cholesterol. Med Lett Drugs Ther 2020; 62:53.

41. KK Ray et al. Safety and efficacy of bempedoic acid to reduce LDL cholesterol. N Engl J Med 2019; 380:1022.

42. AC Goldberg et al. The effect of bempedoic acid vs placebo added to maximally tolerated statins on low-density lipoprotein cholesterol in patients at high risk for cardiovascular disease: the CLEAR Wisdom randomized clinical trial. JAMA 2019; 322:1780.

43. CM Ballantyne et al. Bempedoic acid plus ezetimibe fixed-dose combination in patients with hypercholesterolemia and high CVD risk treated with maximally tolerated statin therapy. Eur J Prev Cardiol 2020; 27:593.

44. Drugs for hypertriglyceridemia. Med Lett Drugs Ther 2013; 55:17.

45. HB Rubins et al. Gemfibrozil for the secondary prevention of coronary heart disease in men with low levels of high-density lipoprotein cholesterol. N Engl J Med 1999; 341:410.

46. P Willeit et al. Baseline and on-statin treatment lipoprotein(a) levels for prediction of cardiovascular events: individual patient-data meta-analysis of statin outcome trials. Lancet 2018; 392:1311.

47. HPS2-THRIVE Collaborative Group. Effects of extended-release niacin with laropiprant in high-risk patients. N Engl J Med 2014; 371:203.

48. FJ Raal et al. Inhibition of PCSK9 with evolocumab in homozygous familial hypercholesterolaemia (TESLA Part B): a randomised, double-blind, placebo-controlled trial. Lancet 2015; 385:341.

49. Two new drugs for homozygous familial hypercholesterolemia. Med Lett Drugs Ther 2013; 55:25.

50. FJ Raal et al. Evinacumab for homozygous familial hypercholesterolemia. N Engl J Med 2020; 383:711.

51. Evinacumab (Evkeeza) for homozygous familial hyper-cholesterolemia. Med Lett Drugs Ther 2021; 63:66.

| Nonopioid Drugs for Pain

Original publication date – March 2022

Nonopioid drugs can be used in the treatment of many nociceptive and neuropathic pain conditions.[1] For severe pain, especially severe chronic cancer pain, use of opioids may be necessary. Noninvasive nonpharmacologic treatments, including physical and psychological therapies, have been shown to improve pain and function in patients with some common chronic pain conditions and are unlikely to cause serious harms.[2] A multimodal approach to analgesic therapy can increase pain control while reducing opioid use and adverse effects.

NONOPIOID ANALGESICS

For initial treatment of mild to moderate pain, nonopioid analgesics such as acetaminophen and nonsteroidal anti-inflammatory drugs (NSAIDs) are preferred.

ACETAMINOPHEN — Acetaminophen is available in multiple oral formulations, often in combination with other over-the-counter (OTC) or prescription drugs, and in rectal and IV formulations. It has no clinically significant anti-inflammatory activity and is generally less effective than an NSAID in relieving pain, but it has fewer adverse effects. In some studies in patients with chronic pain, acetaminophen was not more effective than placebo.[3,4]

Key Points: Treatment of Pain

Acute Pain

► For initial treatment of **mild to moderate** pain, nonopioid analgesics such as acetaminophen and NSAIDs are preferred.

► For **moderate** pain, NSAIDs are more effective than acetaminophen and may be as effective or more effective than oral opioids combined with acetaminophen or even injected opioids.

► For **moderate to severe** pain, a combination of an NSAID and acetaminophen may be as effective as an opioid/acetaminophen combination.

► For **severe** pain, a short-acting full opioid agonist (used in the lowest dosage for the shortest time possible) may be required.[1]

Chronic Noncancer Pain

► Nonpharmacologic therapy can be tried first.

► NSAIDs are generally more effective than acetaminophen, but long-term use can cause gastrointestinal, renal, and cardiovascular toxicity.

► Topical NSAIDs should be considered before oral NSAIDs for localized pain (e.g., hand or knee osteoarthritis pain).

► For severe pain that has not responded to other agents, use of opioids may be necessary.[1]

Chronic Cancer Pain

► Full opioid agonists are generally the drugs of choice for severe pain.[1]

Neuropathic Pain

► For initial treatment, an antidepressant (tricyclic or SNRI) or an antiseizure drug (gabapentin or pregabalin) can be used.

► Combining an antidepressant and an antiseizure drug may have a synergistic analgesic effect.

► Topical agents such as lidocaine or capsaicin can be used for localized pain.

► For severe pain that has not responded to other agents, use of opioids may be necessary.[1]

1. Use of multimodal analgesic therapy can reduce the need for opioids.

Adverse Effects – Most healthy patients can take up to 4 grams of acetaminophen daily with no adverse effects, but repeated use of such doses has been associated with alanine aminotransferase (ALT) and aspartate aminotransferase (AST) elevations. Acetaminophen overdosage can cause serious or fatal hepatotoxicity. In some patients, such as those who are fasting, are heavy alcohol users, or are concurrently taking an interacting drug or herbal supplement, hepatotoxicity can develop after moderate overdosage or even with high therapeutic doses. Acute kidney injury can also occur with acetaminophen overdosage. In patients with hypertension, regular daily intake of 4 grams of acetaminophen increases systolic blood pressure by about 5 mm Hg.[5] Some meta-analyses of cohort and case-control studies have suggested that long-term use of acetaminophen is associated with an increased risk of renal cell cancer.[6]

Drug Interactions – Acetaminophen is metabolized by CYP2E1; concomitant use of drugs that induce CYP2E1, such as carbamazepine, phenobarbital, or isoniazid (INH), can increase concentrations of the hepatotoxic metabolite of acetaminophen. Administration of acetaminophen with drugs that compete for glucuronidation, such as zidovudine, can increase the risk of hepatotoxicity. Continued use of acetaminophen may increase the anticoagulant effect of warfarin (*Coumadin*, and others) in some patients.[7]

Pregnancy – Occasional use of oral acetaminophen during pregnancy is generally considered safe. Some observational studies and meta-analyses have suggested that prenatal exposure to acetaminophen is associated with an increased risk of attention-deficit/hyperactivity disorder (ADHD), autism spectrum disorder, and urogenital disorders in children, but high-quality evidence is lacking.[8]

SALICYLATES — Aspirin is effective for most types of mild to moderate pain, but it is now used mainly in low doses as a platelet inhibitor. Aspirin is available in multiple oral formulations, often in combination with other OTC or prescription drugs.

Unlike other NSAIDs, a single dose of aspirin irreversibly inhibits platelet function for the 8- to 10-day life of the platelet, interfering with hemostasis and prolonging bleeding time. A single dose can precipitate asthma symptoms in aspirin-sensitive patients. High doses or chronic use can cause gastrointestinal (GI) ulceration and salicylate intoxication. Buffered or enteric-coated formulations can reduce the incidence of GI discomfort, but not the risk of GI ulceration. Aspirin should not be used during viral syndromes in children and teenagers because of the risk of Reye's syndrome.

Salsalate and **diflunisal** are nonacetylated salicylates. Salsalate does not interfere with platelet aggregation. Low doses (250 mg twice daily) of diflunisal have no effect on platelets, and the usual dosage of 500 mg twice daily has a minimal effect that is not likely to be clinically significant. These drugs are only rarely associated with GI bleeding, and are well tolerated by asthmatic patients.

NSAIDS — Standard doses of nonselective NSAIDs such as ibuprofen or naproxen are more effective than standard doses of acetaminophen for treatment of moderate acute and chronic pain.[9] In some types of acute pain, NSAIDs have an analgesic effect that is equal to or greater than that of usual doses of an oral opioid combined with acetaminophen.[10] Meta-analyses of randomized trials in patients with chronic low back pain or spinal pain have found that NSAIDs reduce pain intensity and improve disability compared to placebo; the efficacy of different NSAIDs appeared to be similar in these patients.[11,12]

Topical NSAIDs should be considered before oral NSAIDs for treatment of localized pain (e.g., sprains, knee or hand osteoarthritis).[13] Several NSAIDs are available in **IV** formulations (see Table 1). IV ketorolac is frequently used in the emergency department for treatment of moderate to severe pain and post-operatively to reduce opioid use.[14]

Adverse Effects – *Bleeding* – NSAIDs can interfere with platelet function and prolong bleeding time (celecoxib and, to a lesser extent, meloxicam and nabumetone are exceptions). The NSAID-induced antiplatelet effect, unlike that of aspirin, is reversible when the NSAID is cleared.

Gastrointestinal – Dyspepsia and GI ulceration, perforation, and bleeding can occur with all NSAIDs, including parenteral formulations, often without warning. High doses, prolonged use, previous peptic ulcer disease, concomitant use of systemic corticosteroids or aspirin (even

81 mg/day), excessive alcohol intake, and advanced age increase the risk of these complications. Celecoxib causes less GI toxicity than nonselective NSAIDs.[15] The potent NSAID indomethacin is associated with a high risk of GI adverse effects; it should not be used in any dosage for treatment of mild to moderate pain. Use of ketorolac is limited to 5 days because of its high risk of adverse effects, particularly GI toxicity. Taking an NSAID with a proton pump inhibitor such as omeprazole (*Prilosec OTC*, and generics) may decrease the incidence of GI toxicity.

Renal – All NSAIDs, including celecoxib, inhibit renal prostaglandins, decrease renal blood flow, cause fluid retention, and may cause hypertension and renal failure, particularly in elderly patients. Diminished renal function or decreased effective intravascular volume due to diuretic therapy, cirrhosis, or heart failure increases the risk of NSAID-induced renal toxicity.

Cardiovascular – All NSAIDs, especially COX-2 selective NSAIDs such as celecoxib, may have a prothrombotic effect and have been associated with an increased risk of serious cardiovascular events. Among nonselective NSAIDs, the risk appears to be highest with diclofenac and lowest with naproxen.[16,17]

Others – NSAIDs can precipitate asthma symptoms and anaphylactoid reactions in aspirin-sensitive patients. They frequently cause small increases in aminotransferase levels; serious hepatotoxicity is rare, but it may occur more frequently with diclofenac. Pancreatitis has been reported. Cholestatic hepatitis has occurred with celecoxib.

NSAIDs can cause CNS adverse effects such as dizziness, anxiety, drowsiness, confusion, depression, disorientation, severe headache, and aseptic meningitis. They have been associated with both mild and severe skin reactions, including exfoliative dermatitis, Stevens-Johnson syndrome, and toxic epidermal necrolysis. NSAIDs rarely cause blood dyscrasias; aplastic anemia has been reported with ibuprofen, fenoprofen, naproxen, indomethacin, tolmetin, and piroxicam. Long-term use of NSAIDs has been associated with an increased risk of renal cell cancer.[6]

Table 1. Some Nonopioid Analgesics for Pain

Drug	Some Available Formulations
Acetaminophen[3] – generic	325, 500 mg tabs[4] 650 mg ER tabs[4]
Ofirmev (Mallinckrodt)	10 mg/mL IV soln
Salicylates	
Aspirin – generic *Bayer* (Bayer)	325 mg tabs, 500 mg caplets[4,9]
Diflunisal – generic	500 mg tabs
Salsalate – generic	500, 750 mg tabs
Some Nonselective NSAIDs	
Diclofenac[10] – generic	50 mg tabs
Zipsor (Depomed) *Zorvolex* (Iroko)	25 mg caps 35 mg caps
Etodolac – generic	200, 300 mg caps; 400, 500 mg tabs
extended-release – generic[12]	400, 500, 600 mg ER tabs

ER = extended-release; soln = solution
1. Dosage adjustments may be needed for renal or hepatic impairment.
2. Approximate WAC for one week of treatment with the lowest dose and/or longest dosing interval. WAC = wholesaler acquisition cost or manufacturer's published price to wholesalers; WAC represents a published catalogue or list price and may not represent an actual transactional price. Source: AnalySource® Monthly. February 5, 2022. Reprinted with permission by First Databank, Inc. All rights reserved. ©2022. www.fdbhealth.com/policies/drug-pricing-policy.
3. Acetaminophen is included in multiple prescription and OTC products for treatment of pain, cough, cold, flu, migraine, insomnia, etc., increasing the risk for accidental overdosage.
4. Also available in other strengths and dosage forms, alone and in combination with other drugs, both OTC and by prescription. Amount in prescription combination products is limited to 325 mg/dosage unit.
5. Cost at www.walgreens.com. Accessed February 17, 2022.

Usual Adult Analgesic Dosage[1]	Comments	Cost[2]
650 mg q4-6h or 1000 mg q6h	▸ Generally less effective than NSAIDs	$1.70[5]
1300 mg q8h (max 4000 mg/day)		1.50[5]
<50 kg: 15 mg/kg q6h or 12.5 mg/kg q4h (max 75 mg/kg/day)	▸ Time to pain relief: 27 minutes[6]	189.50[7,8]
≥50 kg: 1000 mg q6h or 650 mg q4h (max 4000 mg/day)		
325-650 mg q4-6h (max 4000 mg/day)		0.30[5]
		2.20[5]
500 mg q8-12h (max 1500 mg/day)	▸ 500 mg comparable to 650 mg of acetaminophen or aspirin with slower onset and longer duration	23.10
500 mg q6h or 1000 mg q12h (max 3000 mg/day)		8.40
50 mg q8-12h (max 200 mg/day)	▸ Comparable to aspirin with longer duration	6.30
25 mg qid (max 200 mg/day)		434.60
35 mg tid		183.10
200-400 mg q6-8h (max 1000 mg/day)[11]	▸ 200 mg comparable to ibuprofen 400 mg; possibly superior to aspirin 650 mg	2.20
400-1000 mg once/day		1.40

6. Med Lett Drugs Ther 2020; 62:100.
7. Cost based on treatment of a 70-kg patient.
8. Cost for one day of treatment at the lowest dosage.
9. Also available in chewable, buffered, enteric-coated, and extended-release formulations.
10. Also available in enteric-coated and extended-release tabs for use in osteoarthritis, rheumatoid arthritis, and ankylosing spondylitis, and topically as a patch (*Flector*, and generics) for treatment of pain due to minor strains, sprains, and contusions, as a topical gel (*Voltaren Arthritis Pain 1% Gel*; available OTC) for use in osteoarthritis, and as a 1.5% solution and a 2% solution (*Pennsaid 2%*) for use in osteoarthritis of the knee. Also available in a fixed-dose combination with misoprostol (*Arthrotec*) to decrease GI toxicity (contraindicated in pregnant women).
11. For use in osteoarthritis or rheumatoid arthritis the dosage is 300 mg bid or tid, 400 mg bid, or 500 mg bid.
12. FDA-approved only for use in osteoarthritis and rheumatoid arthritis.

Continued on next page

Table 1. Some Nonopioid Analgesics for Pain (continued)

Drug	Some Available Formulations
Some Nonselective NSAIDs (continued)	
Fenoprofen − generic	200, 400 mg caps; 600 mg tabs
Nalfon (Xspire)	400 mg caps
Flurbiprofen[11] − generic	100 mg tabs
Ibuprofen[15] − generic	400, 600, 800 mg tabs
Caldolor (Cumberland)	100 mg/mL IV soln
Ibuprofen OTC − generic *Advil* (GSK Consumer)	100, 200 mg tabs; 200 mg caps
Ketoprofen − generic	50, 75 mg caps
extended-release − generic	200 mg ER caps
Ketorolac − generic	10 mg tabs
	15 mg/mL, 30 mg/mL, 60 mg/2 mL injection
Sprix (Egalet)	15.75 mg/intranasal spray

ER = extended-release; soln = solution
13. For use in osteoarthritis or rheumatoid arthritis, the dosage is 400-600 mg tid or qid.
14. Cost for one week of treatment with 400 mg tid.
15. Also available in a fixed-dose combination with famotidine (*Duexis*) to decrease GI toxicity.
16. Recommended only for continuation therapy after IM or IV ketorolac; total duration not to exceed 5 days.
17. Cost of 5 days' treatment.

Usual Adult Analgesic Dosage[1]	Comments	Cost[2]
200 mg q4-6h (max 3200 mg/day)[13]		$355.80
		109.20[14]
100 mg q12h (max 300 mg/day)		8.00
400 mg q4-6h (max 2400 mg/day)	► 200 mg equal to 650 mg of aspirin or acetaminophen; 400 mg comparable to acetaminophen/codeine	1.20
400-800 mg IV q6h (max 3200 mg/day)	► Time to pain relief: 15-30 minutes[6]	38.60[7]
200-400 mg q4-6h (max 1200 mg/day)	► 200 mg equal to 650 mg of aspirin or acetaminophen	1.10[5] 2.20[5]
50 mg q6h or 75 mg q8h (max 300 mg/day) 200 mg once/day	► 25 mg comparable to ibuprofen 400 mg and superior to aspirin 650 mg; 50 mg superior to acetaminophen/ codeine	33.60 60.60
10 mg q4-6h (max 40 mg/day)[16]	► 10 mg comparable to ibuprofen 400 or 800 mg or naproxen 500-550 mg	13.60[17]
<65 yrs: 30 mg IM or IV q6h (max 120 mg/day)[18] ≥65 yrs: 15 mg IM or IV q6h (max 60 mg/day)[18]	► Comparable to 12 mg IM morphine with longer duration ► Time to pain relief: 30 minutes[6]	31.80[19]
<65 yrs: 1 spray q6-8h in each nostril (max 126 mg/day)[20] ≥65 yrs: 1 spray q6-8h in one nostril (max 63 mg/day)[20]		2245.90[21]

18. Total duration not to exceed 5 days because of adverse effects; can also be given IM as a single 60-mg (<65 years) or 30-mg (≥65 years) dose.
19. Cost of 5 days' treatment for a <65-year-old patient.
20. Dose in patients weighing <50 kg or with renal impairment (GFR 30-90 mL/min) is one spray in one nostril; maximum 4 doses/day for up to 5 days.
21. Cost of one carton containing 5 single-day nasal spray bottles.

Continued on next page

Table 1. Some Nonopioid Analgesics for Pain (continued)

Drug	Some Available Formulations
Some Nonselective NSAIDs (continued)	
Meclofenamate – generic	50, 100 mg caps
Mefenamic acid – generic	250 mg caps
Meloxicam – generic	7.5, 15 mg tabs; 7.5 mg/5 mL PO susp
Mobic (Boehringer Ingelheim)[11]	7.5, 15 mg tabs
submicronized – generic[23]	5, 10 mg caps
Anjeso (Baudax Bio)	30 mg/mL vials
Nabumetone[12] – generic	500, 750 mg tabs
Naproxen – generic	250, 375, 500 mg tabs; 375, 500 mg enteric-coated tabs; 25 mg/mL PO susp
Naprosyn, EC-Naprosyn (Canton, Athena)	500 mg tabs; 375, 500 mg enteric-coated tabs; 25 mg/mL PO susp
Naproxen sodium[26] – generic	275, 550 mg tabs
Anaprox DX (Canton)	550 mg tabs
Naproxen sodium OTC –	
generic	220 mg tabs, caps
Aleve (Bayer)	

susp = suspension
22. Duration of use usually not to exceed 1 week for acute pain or 2-3 days for dysmenorrhea.
23. FDA-approved only for use in osteoarthritis.
24. IV bolus given over 15 seconds.

Usual Adult Analgesic Dosage[1]	Comments	Cost[2]
50-100 mg q4h (max 400 mg/day)		$140.10
500 mg once, then 250 mg q6h[22] (max 1250 mg on day 1, then 1000 mg/day)	► Comparable to aspirin but more effective than aspirin in dysmenorrhea	404.30
7.5-15 mg once/day 5 or 10 mg once/day	► Appears to be more selective for COX-2 than COX-1 at low doses (7.5 mg)	0.30 67.80 173.90
30 mg IV q24h[24]	► Time to pain relief: 2-3 hours; slower than other nonopioid IV analgesics[6]	282.00[25]
500 or 750 mg q8-12h (max 2000 mg/day)		4.10
250 mg q6-8h or 500 mg q12h (max 1250 mg on day 1, then 1000 mg/day)	► 250 mg probably comparable to aspirin 650 mg with longer duration; 500 mg superior to aspirin 650 mg	1.50 83.00
275 mg q6-8h or 550 mg q12h (max 1375 mg on day 1, then 1100 mg/day)	► 275 mg comparable to aspirin 650 mg with longer duration; 550 mg comparable to 400 mg ibuprofen with longer duration	4.40 130.30
220 mg q8-12h (max 660 mg/day)		1.00[5] 1.40[5]

25. Cost of 3 days' treatment.
26. Also available in a fixed-dose combination with esomeprazole (*Vimovo*, and generics) to decrease GI toxicity.

Continued on next page

Table 1. Some Nonopioid Analgesics for Pain (continued)	
Drug	**Some Available Formulations**
Selective COX-2 Inhibitor	
Celecoxib[27] – generic *Celebrex* (Pfizer)	50, 100, 200, 400 mg caps

27. Also available in an oral solution *(Elyxyb)* for acute treatment of migraine.
28. The dosage is 200 mg/day for use in osteoarthritis and 200-400 mg/day for use in rheumatoid arthritis.

Pregnancy – Exposure to NSAIDs around the time of conception or during pregnancy has been associated with an increased risk of miscarriage,[18] but the data are weak. In 2020, the FDA required a new warning in the labels of prescription and OTC NSAID-containing products advising against their use during pregnancy beginning at 20 weeks' gestation because of a risk of fetal renal dysfunction that could lead to low amniotic fluid levels (oligohydramnios) and neonatal renal impairment. NSAID labels had already warned against use of the drugs beginning at 30 weeks' gestation because of the risk of premature closure of the fetal ductus arteriosus.[19]

Drug Interactions – NSAIDs can decrease the effectiveness of diuretics, beta blockers, ACE inhibitors, and some other antihypertensive drugs. They can increase serum concentrations of lithium and methotrexate, possibly resulting in toxicity. NSAIDs may increase the INR in patients taking warfarin. Patients taking aspirin for cardiovascular protection should not take ibuprofen or naproxen regularly because they can interfere with aspirin's antiplatelet effect. Celecoxib is a moderate CYP2D6 inhibitor; it can increase serum concentrations of CYP2D6 substrates. Celecoxib, diclofenac, flurbiprofen, ibuprofen, indomethacin, meloxicam, naproxen, and piroxicam are CYP2C9 substrates; dosage reductions may be required in CYP2C9 poor metabolizers and patients taking a CYP2C9 inhibitor.[20]

Usual Adult Analgesic Dosage[1]	Comments	Cost[2]
400 mg once, then 200 mg q12h (max 600 mg on day 1, then 400 mg/day)[28]	► Comparable to naproxen or ibuprofen	$4.50 195.00

COMBINATION TREATMENT FOR ACUTE PAIN — For treatment of moderate to severe acute pain, a combination of an NSAID and acetaminophen is more effective than either drug alone and may be an alternative to opioid analgesics. In a double-blind trial, 411 patients with moderate to severe acute extremity pain were randomized to receive single doses of one of four combination analgesic regimens: ibuprofen 400 mg plus acetaminophen 1000 mg, or either oxycodone 5 mg, hydrocodone 5 mg, or codeine 30 mg plus acetaminophen 300-325 mg. There were no statistically significant differences in pain reduction between the nonopioid regimen and the opioid-containing regimens at two hours post-dose.[21]

ADJUVANT PAIN MEDICATIONS

For initial treatment of neuropathic pain, a tricyclic antidepressant (TCA), a serotonin and norepinephrine reuptake inhibitor (SNRI), or an antiseizure drug can be used.

TCAs — **Amitriptyline**, **nortriptyline**, and **imipramine** have been shown to relieve many types of neuropathic pain, including diabetic neuropathy, postherpetic neuralgia, polyneuropathy, and nerve injury or infiltration with cancer.[22] The analgesic effects of these drugs are likely due to their inhibition of norepinephrine and serotonin reuptake.

Table 2. Some Adjuvant Pain Medications[1]

Drug	Some Available Formulations
Tricyclic Antidepressants	
Amitriptyline – generic	10, 25, 50, 75, 100, 150 mg tabs
Imipramine HCl – generic	10, 25, 50 mg tabs
Imipramine pamoate – generic	75, 100, 125, 150 mg caps
Nortriptyline – generic	10, 25, 50, 75 mg caps; 10 mg/5 mL PO soln
Pamelor (Mallinckrodt)	10, 25, 50, 75 mg caps
Serotonin and Norepinephrine Reuptake Inhibitors (SNRIs)	
Venlafaxine – generic	25, 37.5, 50, 75, 100 mg tabs
extended-release – generic	37.5, 75, 150 tabs and caps; 225 mg tabs
Effexor XR (Pfizer)	37.5, 75, 150 mg caps
Duloxetine – generic	20, 30, 60 mg delayed-release caps
Cymbalta (Lilly)	
Milnacipran – Savella (Allergan)	12.5, 25, 50, 100 mg tabs
Antiseizure Drugs	
Gabapentin – generic	100, 300, 400 mg caps; 600, 800 mg tabs;
Neurontin (Pfizer)	250 mg/5 mL PO soln
extended-release	
Gralise (Depomed)	300, 600 mg ER tabs
Horizant (Azurity)	300, 600 mg ER tabs
Pregabalin – generic	25, 50, 75, 100, 150, 200, 225, 300 mg caps;
Lyrica (Pfizer)	20 mg/mL PO soln
extended-release – generic	82.5, 165, 330 mg ER tabs
Lyrica CR	
Carbamazepine – generic	200 mg tabs; 100 mg chewable tabs;
Tegretol (Novartis)	100 mg/5 mL PO susp
extended-release – generic	100, 200 mg ER caps and tabs; 300 mg ER caps; 400 mg ER tabs
Tegretol XR (Novartis)	100, 200, 400 mg ER tabs
Carbatrol (Takeda)	100, 200, 300 mg ER caps
Equetro (Validus)	100, 200, 300 mg ER caps

ER = extended-release
1. Some of the drugs listed here are not FDA-approved for treatment of pain.
2. Dosage adjustments may be needed for renal or hepatic impairment.
3. Approximate WAC for 30 days' treatment at the lowest usual dosage and/or longest dosing interval. WAC = wholesaler acquisition cost or manufacturer's published price to wholesalers; WAC represents a published catalogue or list price and may not represent an actual transactional price. Source: AnalySource® Monthly. February 5, 2022. Reprinted with permission by First Databank, Inc. All rights reserved. ©2022. www.fdbhealth.com/policies/drug-pricing-policy.

Usual Dosage for Pain[2]	Cost[3]
25-100 mg once/day	$6.60
50-100 mg once/day or divided	9.30
75-100 mg once/day	354.00
75 mg once/day or divided	13.50
	1249.60
75 mg once/day-tid	7.20
75-150 mg once/day	9.30
	487.80
60 mg once/day	9.00
	272.40
50 mg bid	442.10
600-1200 mg bid	9.00
	700.20
1800 mg once/day	864.60
600 mg bid	904.40
75-300 mg bid or 50-200 mg tid	7.80
	515.40
330-660 mg once/day	265.60
	442.70
100-600 mg bid	22.80
	75.90
100-600 mg bid	55.20
	81.60
	106.40
	231.60

Continued on next page

Table 2. Some Adjuvant Pain Medications[1] (continued)	
Drug	**Some Available Formulations**
Antiseizure Drugs (continued)	
Oxcarbazepine – generic	150, 300, 600 mg tabs; 300 mg/5 mL PO susp
Trileptal (Novartis)	
extended-release –	
Oxtellar XR (Supernus)	150, 300, 600 mg ER tabs

TCAs commonly cause orthostatic hypotension, weight gain, sedation, sexual dysfunction, and anticholinergic effects (e.g., urinary retention, constipation, dry mouth, blurred vision, memory impairment, confusion).

SNRIs – Duloxetine is FDA-approved for treatment of diabetic peripheral neuropathy pain, fibromyalgia, and chronic musculoskeletal pain. In patients with chronic low back pain or osteoarthritis, it has been only modestly more effective than placebo.[23] In one open-label, randomized trial in 132 patients with chronic osteoarthritis of the hip and/or knee, addition of duloxetine 60 mg/day to usual care (mainly acetaminophen or NSAIDs) was not more effective in reducing pain than usual care alone.[24] **Venlafaxine** has been effective in various types of neuropathic pain, including diabetic neuropathy, post-mastectomy pain syndrome, and chemotherapy-induced neurotoxicity, and has also been used to treat fibromyalgia,[25] but it is not FDA-approved for any of these indications. **Milnacipran**, which is FDA-approved only for use in fibromyalgia, is moderately effective in decreasing pain and improving function.[26] It inhibits norepinephrine reuptake to a greater extent than it does serotonin reuptake. How it compares to duloxetine or venlafaxine is unclear.

SNRIs can cause nausea, dizziness, increased sweating, tachycardia, constipation, urinary retention, and a dose-dependent increase in blood pressure. Severe discontinuation symptoms and sustained hypertension can occur with venlafaxine. Severe liver injury has been reported with duloxetine and milnacipran.[27]

Usual Dosage for Pain[2]	Cost[3]
300-600 mg bid	$33.60
	496.80
600-2400 mg once/day	613.20

ANTISEIZURE DRUGS — In controlled trials, **gabapentin** has been effective in reducing pain associated with postherpetic neuralgia (an FDA-approved use) and diabetic neuropathy.[28] **Pregabalin**, which is structurally similar to gabapentin, is FDA-approved for treatment of postherpetic neuralgia and diabetic peripheral neuropathy.[29] The immediate-release formulation is also approved for treatment of fibromyalgia (the extended-release formulation was not effective for this indication).

In a randomized, double-blind, 8-week trial in 209 patients with acute or chronic sciatica, pregabalin 150-600 mg daily did not significantly reduce the intensity of leg pain compared to placebo.[30]

Gabapentin and pregabalin can cause dizziness, somnolence, peripheral edema, and weight gain. In 2019, the FDA required new warnings in the labels of both gabapentin and pregabalin about a risk of life-threatening or fatal respiratory depression in patients with respiratory risk factors (e.g., chronic obstructive pulmonary disease [COPD], concurrent use of opioids or other CNS depressants). Elderly patients are at increased risk.[31]

Routine use of gabapentin and pregabalin can lead to physical dependence. Use of higher-than-recommended doses to achieve euphoric highs is increasingly being reported.[32] Pregabalin is a schedule V controlled substance. Gabapentin is classified as a schedule V controlled substance in some states.

Carbamazepine is FDA-approved for treatment of pain associated with trigeminal neuralgia, but it can rarely cause serious adverse effects such as aplastic anemia, agranulocytosis, and toxic epidermal necrolysis. **Oxcarbazepine**, which is not FDA-approved for treatment of pain, has been shown to be modestly effective in relieving peripheral neuropathic pain and may be tolerated better than carbamazepine.[33]

COMBINATION TREATMENT FOR NEUROPATHIC PAIN — Combining an antidepressant and an anti-seizure drug may produce a synergistic analgesic effect in neuropathic pain syndromes, but clinical trials have produced conflicting results and high-quality evidence is lacking.[34]

OTHER DRUGS — **Ziconotide** *(Prialt)*, a synthetic neuronal N-type calcium channel blocker, is administered intrathecally via a programmable microinfusion device for treatment of severe chronic pain. It has been effective, both as monotherapy and when added to standard therapy, for treatment of refractory severe chronic pain, including neuropathic pain. Unlike opioids, ziconotide does not cause tolerance, dependence, or respiratory depression, and it is not a controlled substance.[35] Elevations in creatine kinase levels are common and severe psychiatric effects (e.g., paranoid reactions, psychosis) and CNS toxicity (e.g., confusion, somnolence, unresponsiveness) can occur.[36]

Caffeine in doses of 65-200 mg may enhance the analgesic effect of acetaminophen, aspirin, or ibuprofen in patients with acute pain.[37] A fixed-dose combination of the skeletal muscle relaxant **orphenadrine citrate**, aspirin, and caffeine *(Orphengesic Forte*; previously available as *Norgesic Forte)* is now available with a prescription for treatment of mild to moderate pain caused by acute musculoskeletal disorders.[38] Comparative trials with less expensive nonopioid analgesics are lacking.

Corticosteroids can produce analgesia in some patients with inflammatory diseases or tumor infiltration of nerves. In small trials, treatment with **low-dose naltrexone** (typically 4.5 mg/day) has improved symptoms in patients with multiple sclerosis and other chronic pain disorders.[39] Oral and transdermal patch formulations of the alpha$_2$-adrenergic agonist **clonidine** may improve pain and hyperalgesia in sympathetically maintained pain, but clonidine can cause hypotension. Injections of **botulinum toxin type A** have been shown to be effective for treatment of postherpetic neuralgia, diabetic neuropathy, trigeminal neuralgia, and intractable neuropathic pain such as poststroke pain and spinal cord injury.[40] IV infusions of the anesthetic agent **ketamine** appear to provide short-term improvements in some patients with complex regional pain syndrome, neuropathic pain, and other refractory chronic pain conditions, but high-quality evidence is lacking.[41]

Randomized trials of **cannabinoids** have found some evidence of efficacy for second-line treatment of cancer pain, neuropathic pain, and the spasticity of multiple sclerosis. Results of randomized controlled trials suggest that **cannabis** may alleviate neuropathic pain over the short term in some patients; the efficacy of cannabis for other types of chronic pain remains to be established.[42]

Topical Analgesics – Two **lidocaine** patches *(Lidoderm 5%, ZTlido 1.8%)*, available by prescription, are FDA-approved for treatment of postherpetic neuralgia.[43] Lidocaine 4% patches are available OTC. An 8% **capsaicin** patch *(Qutenza)* is FDA-approved for treatment of postherpetic neuralgia and diabetic peripheral neuropathy of the feet. Application of the patch for one hour for postherpetic neuralgia or for 30 minutes for peripheral neuropathy has been modestly effective in reducing pain for up to 3 months.[44,45] Lower-strength cream and patch formulations of capsaicin are available OTC.

1. NB Finnerup. Nonnarcotic methods of pain management. N Engl J Med 2019; 380:2440.
2. AC Skelly et al. Noninvasive nonpharmacological treatment for chronic pain: a systematic review update [internet]. Rockville (MD): Agency for Healthcare Research and Quality (US); 2020 Apr. Report No.: 20-EHC009. Available at: https://bit.ly/3uwrh33. Accessed February 17, 2022.
3. BT Saragiotto et al. Paracetamol for low back pain. Cochrane Database Syst Rev 2016; 6:CD012230.
4. BR da Costa et al. Effectiveness and safety of non-steroidal anti-inflammatory drugs and opioid treatment for knee and hip osteoarthritis: network meta-analysis. BMJ 2021; 375:n2321.

Nonopioid Drugs for Pain

5. IM MacIntyre et al. Regular acetaminophen use and blood pressure in people with hypertension: the PATH-BP trial. Circulation 2022; 145:416.

6. TK Choueiri et al. Analgesic use and the risk of kidney cancer: a meta-analysis of epidemiologic studies. Int J Cancer 2014; 134:384.

7. Addendum: Warfarin-acetaminophen interaction. Med Lett Drugs Ther 2008; 50:45.

8. S Alwan et al. Paracetamol use in pregnancy – caution over causal inference from available data. Nat Rev Endocrinol 2021 Dec 14 (epub).

9. RA Moore et al. Overview review: comparative efficacy of oral ibuprofen and paracetamol (acetaminophen) across acute and chronic pain conditions. Eur J Pain 2015; 19:1213.

10. SA Cooper et al. Analgesic efficacy of naproxen sodium versus hydrocodone/ acetaminophen in acute postsurgical dental pain: a randomized, double-blind, placebo-controlled trial. Postgrad Med 2021 Dec 8 (epub).

11. WTM Enthoven et al. Non-steroidal anti-inflammatory drugs for chronic low back pain. Cochrane Database Syst Rev 2016; 2:CD012087.

12. GC Machado et al. Non-steroidal anti-inflammatory drugs for spinal pain: a systematic review and meta-analysis. Ann Rheum Dis 2017; 76:1269.

13. Drugs for osteoarthritis. Med Lett Drugs Ther 2020; 62:57.

14. S Motov et al. Comparison of intravenous ketorolac at three single-dose regimens for treating acute pain in the emergency department: a randomized controlled trial. Ann Emerg Med 2017; 70:177.

15. FKL Chan et al. Gastrointestinal safety of celecoxib versus naproxen in patients with cardiothrombotic diseases and arthritis after upper gastrointestinal bleeding (CONCERN): an industry-independent, double-blind, double-dummy, randomised trial. Lancet 2017; 389:2375.

16. FDA Drug Safety Communication: FDA strengthens warning that non-aspirin nonsteroidal anti-inflammatory drugs (NSAIDs) can cause heart attacks or strokes. July 9, 2015. Available at: https://bit.ly/3gLeYYD. Accessed February 17, 2022.

17. Celecoxib safety revisited. Med Lett Drugs Ther 2016; 58:159.

18. DK Li et al. Use of nonsteroidal antiinflammatory drugs during pregnancy and the risk of miscarriage. Am J Obstet Gynecol 2018; 219:275.

19. In Brief: New warnings on NSAID use in pregnancy. Med Lett Drugs Ther 2020; 62:175.

20. Inhibitors and inducers of CYP enzymes, P-glycoprotein, and other transporters. Med Lett Drugs Ther 2021 October 20 (epub). Available at: medicalletter.org/downloads/ CYP_PGP_Tables.pdf.

21. AK Chang et al. Effect of a single dose of oral opioid and nonopioid analgesics on acute extremity pain in the emergency department: a randomized clinical trial. JAMA 2017; 318:1661.

22. A Liampas et al. Pharmacological management of painful peripheral neuropathies: a systematic review. Pain Ther 2021; 10:55.

23. C Weng et al. Efficacy and safety of duloxetine in osteoarthritis or chronic low back pain: a systematic review and meta-analysis. Osteoarthritis Cartilage 2020; 28:721.

24. JJ van den Driest et al. No added value of duloxetine for patients with chronic pain due to hip or knee osteoarthritis: a cluster randomized trial. Arthritis Rheumatol 2022 January 6 (epub).

25. R Aiyer et al. Treatment of neuropathic pain with venlafaxine: a systematic review. Pain Med 2017; 18:1999.

26. H Gupta et al. Milnacipran for the treatment of fibromyalgia. Health Psychol Res 2021; 9:25532.

27. NB Finnerup et al. Pharmacotherapy for neuropathic pain in adults: a systematic review and meta-analysis. Lancet Neurol 2015; 14:162.

28. N Majdinasab et al. A comparative double-blind randomized study on the effectiveness of duloxetine and gabapentin on painful diabetic peripheral neuropathy. Drug Des Devel Ther 2019; 13:1985.

29. S Derry et al. Pregabalin for neuropathic pain in adults. Cochrane Database Syst Rev 2019; 1:CD007076.

30. S Mathieson et al. Trial of pregabalin for acute and chronic sciatica. N Engl J Med 2017; 376:1111.

31. In Brief: Respiratory depression with gabapentinoids. Med Lett Drugs Ther 2020; 62:81.

32. KE Evoy et al. Abuse and misuse of pregabalin and gabapentin: a systematic review update. Drugs 2021; 81:125.

33. M Zhou et al. Oxcarbazepine for neuropathic pain. Cochrane Database Syst Rev 2017; 12:CD007963.

34. AS Afonso et al. Combination therapy for neuropathic pain: a review of recent evidence. J Clin Med 2021; 10:3533.

35. Ziconotide (Prialt) for chronic pain. Med Lett Drugs Ther 2005; 47:103.

36. TR Deer et al. Intrathecal therapy for chronic pain: a review of morphine and ziconotide as firstline options. Pain Med 2019; 20:784.

37. CJ Derry et al. Caffeine as an analgesic adjuvant for acute pain in adults. Cochrane Database Syst Rev 2014; 12:CD009281.

38. Orphengesic Forte – an old analgesic combination returns. Med Lett Drugs Ther 2020; 62:180.

39. DK Patten et al. The safety and efficacy of low-dose naltrexone in the management of chronic pain and inflammation in multiple sclerosis, fibromyalgia, Crohn's disease, and other chronic pain disorders. Pharmacotherapy 2018; 38:382.

40. J Park and HJ Park. Botulinum toxin for the treatment of neuropathic pain. Toxins (Basel) 2017; 9:260.

41. SP Cohen et al. Consensus guidelines on the use of intravenous ketamine infusions for chronic pain from the American Society of Regional Anesthesia and Pain Medicine, the American Academy of Pain Medicine, and the American Society of Anesthesiologists. Reg Anesth Pain Med 2018; 43:521.

42. Cannabis and cannabinoids. Med Lett Drugs Ther 2019; 61:179.

43. ZTlido – a new lidocaine patch for postherpetic neuralgia. Med Lett Drugs 2019; 61:41.

44. Capsaicin patch (Qutenza) for postherpetic neuralgia. Med Lett Drugs Ther 2011; 53:42.

45. DM Simpson et al. Capsaicin 8% patch in painful diabetic peripheral neuropathy: a randomized, double-blind, placebo-controlled study. J Pain 2017; 18:42.

| Opioids for Pain

Original publication date – December 2022

A new CDC guideline for prescribing opioids for pain recently became available.[1] Nonopioid drugs for pain were reviewed in a previous issue.[2]

ACUTE PAIN — For many types of moderate to severe acute pain, acetaminophen and/or an NSAID may be as effective as an opioid.[3,4] Use of caffeine as a co-analgesic may provide some additional pain relief.[5] If nonopioid drugs and nonpharmacologic treatment (e.g., heat or ice, rest, elevation, immobilization, physical therapy) provide insufficient relief, an immediate-release formulation of a full opioid agonist may be used as needed (i.e., not around the clock) at the lowest effective dose and for the shortest possible duration. Use of extended-release or long-acting opioid formulations initially and for treatment durations >1 week have been associated with overdose and unintended long-term use.[6-8]

CHRONIC PAIN — Use of opioids for treatment of chronic noncancer pain is controversial; evidence of their long-term effectiveness from controlled trials is limited and serious adverse effects can occur.[9-11] As with acute pain, nonopioid drugs and nonpharmacologic therapy may be as effective as an opioid for many types of chronic pain.[12] Full opioid agonists are recommended for treatment of severe chronic cancer pain.

DOSAGE — Opioid dosage requirements vary widely among patients. In general, experts recommend starting with the lowest available strength of an immediate-release opioid and titrating to analgesic effect; for opioid-naive patients, it would be reasonable to start with 5-10 mg of oral morphine per dose (or its equivalent) or 20-30 mg per day (see MME conversion factors in Table 2). After initial titration with an immediate-release opioid, an extended-release or long-acting formulation can be used in patients with continuous severe pain.

ADVERSE EFFECTS — Sedation, dizziness, nausea, vomiting, pruritus, sweating, and constipation are the most common adverse effects of opioids; respiratory depression is the most serious. Tolerance to the respiratory depressant effect develops with chronic use. Administered in usual doses, opioids, including buprenorphine and mixed agonist/antagonists, may decrease respiratory drive and cause apnea in opioid-naive patients, particularly those who are taking other CNS depressants or have COPD, cor pulmonale, decreased respiratory reserve, or pre-existing respiratory depression.

Tolerance usually develops rapidly to the sedative and emetic effects of opioids, but not to constipation; a stimulant or osmotic laxative with or without a stool softener should be started early in treatment. Three oral, peripherally-acting mu-opioid receptor antagonists — methylnaltrexone *(Relistor)*, naloxegol *(Movantik)*, and naldemedine *(Symproic)* — are available for treatment of opioid-induced constipation. They appear to be similar in efficacy and safety, but no direct comparisons are available.[13-15] Lubiprostone *(Amitiza*, and generics), an oral chloride channel activator, may be less effective.[16]

Opioid-induced hyperalgesia has been reported in some patients treated with high doses of opioids. These patients experience worsening pain that cannot be overcome by increasing the dose, but rather by reducing the dose, discontinuing the opioid, or switching to another opioid.[17]

Chronic use of opioids can increase prolactin levels and decrease levels of sex hormones, resulting in reduced sexual function, decreased libido, infertility, mood disturbances, and bone loss.[18] Adrenal insufficiency has

Table 1. Opioid Prescribing for Noncancer Pain[1,2]
► Nonpharmacologic therapy and nonopioid drugs are preferred.
► For acute pain, opioids should be taken as needed rather than around the clock.
► Opioid treatment of subacute noncancer pain (duration 1-3 months) and chronic noncancer pain (duration >3 months) should be combined with nonpharmacologic therapy and nonopioid drugs.
► Immediate-release formulations are recommended for initial opioid treatment; the lowest effective dose should be used, and the quantity prescribed should not exceed the expected amount needed.
► Extended-release or long-acting opioids should be reserved for patients with severe, continuous pain.
► Benefits and risks should be evaluated within 1-4 weeks of starting treatment or of dose escalation, and at least every 3 months with continued treatment. If benefits no longer outweigh risks, other treatments should be optimized and opioids should be tapered to a lower dosage or tapered and discontinued.
► Higher opioid doses are associated with increased risks for motor vehicle injury, opioid use disorder, and overdose. Many patients do not experience benefit from increasing the dose to >50 oral morphine milligram equivalents (MMEs)/day.
► Caution is recommended when opioids are prescribed concurrently with other CNS depressants, especially benzodiazepines.
► The opioid antagonist naloxone should be offered to patients at risk of opioid overdose.
► Buprenorphine or methadone should be prescribed for patients who develop opioid use disorder.
► State prescription drug monitoring program data can be used to determine whether a patient is receiving opioid dosages or combination treatments that increase the risk for overdose.
► Urine drug testing is recommended before starting treatment and at least annually thereafter to assess for use of other controlled prescription drugs and/or illicit drugs.
1. D Dowell et al. MMWR Recomm Rep 2022; 71:1. 2. L Manchikanti et al. Pain Physician 2017; 20(2S):S3.

been reported, typically after >1 month of opioid use.[19] Sleep apnea, depression, falls, and urinary outflow obstruction can also occur.

TOLERANCE — Tolerance develops with chronic use of opioids; the patient first notices a reduction in adverse effects and a shorter duration of analgesia, followed by a decrease in the effectiveness of each dose. It can usually be surmounted and adequate analgesia restored by increasing the dose or by switching to a different opioid. Tolerance to most of the adverse effects of opioids (except constipation) develops at least as rapidly as tolerance to the analgesic effect.

Cross-tolerance exists among all full opioid agonists, but it is incomplete; when switching to another opioid, reducing the equianalgesic dose by at least 25-50% is recommended (see MME conversion factors in Table 2). Switching opioid-tolerant patients to methadone may improve pain relief, but should be done cautiously by an experienced clinician; the equianalgesic dose of methadone is not well-established in opioid-tolerant patients.

DEPENDENCE — Clinically significant physical dependence can begin to develop after several days of continued treatment with an opioid. Withdrawal symptoms will occur if the drug is discontinued suddenly or an opioid antagonist or partial agonist is given. Opioids should be tapered gradually to reduce withdrawal symptoms.

DRUG INTERACTIONS — Use of opioids with alcohol, general anesthetics, phenothiazines, sedative-hypnotics such as benzodiazepines or barbiturates, tricyclic anti-depressants, first-generation antihistamines, muscle relaxants, gabapentinoids, or other CNS depressants increases the risk of respiratory depression and death. Concurrent use of an opioid and an anticholinergic drug can cause urinary retention and severe constipation, possibly leading to paralytic ileus. Use of opioids with serotonergic drugs has resulted in serotonin syndrome, especially with fentanyl, meperidine, methadone, tapentadol, and tramadol.[20] Use of an opioid with or within 14 days of a monoamine oxidase (MAO) inhibitor can cause serotonin syndrome or opioid toxicity and is not recommended.

Buprenorphine, fentanyl, hydrocodone, meperidine, methadone, oliceridine, oxycodone, and tramadol are metabolized at least partly by CYP3A4. Concurrent use of a drug that inhibits CYP3A4 (or discontinuation of a CYP3A4 inducer) can increase serum concentrations of these opioids and the risk of sedation and respiratory depression. Concurrent use of a drug that induces CYP3A4 (or discontinuation of a CYP3A4 inhibitor) could decrease their serum concentrations and analgesic effect, possibly leading to withdrawal symptoms. Concomitant use of methadone with CYP2B6, 2C19, 2C9, or 2D6 inhibitors (or discontinuation of inducers of these isozymes) may increase methadone serum concentrations. CYP2D6 inhibitors can decrease the analgesic effect of codeine and tramadol.[21]

Opioids delay gastric emptying and the absorption of orally administered drugs, including the $P2Y_{12}$ platelet inhibitors clopidogrel, prasugrel, and ticagrelor. Use of morphine has been associated with an increased risk of recurrent ischemia, myocardial infarction, and death in patients taking clopidogrel after an acute coronary syndrome.[22,23]

Cimetidine can potentiate the effects of morphine. P-glycoprotein inhibitors such as amiodarone can increase morphine exposure.[21]

PREGNANCY — Opioid use during pregnancy has been associated with preterm delivery, poor fetal growth, stillbirth, birth defects (e.g., neural tube defects, congenital heart defects, gastroschisis), poor physiological development, and neurodevelopmental disorders.[24,25] It can also lead to neonatal opioid withdrawal syndrome. Opioid withdrawal during pregnancy has been associated with spontaneous abortion and premature labor. Pregnant women who are physically dependent on opioids should receive buprenorphine or methadone.[26]

OVERDOSE REVERSAL – Administration of an opioid antagonist can reverse severe respiratory depression due to an opioid overdose.

Naloxone is the opioid antagonist of choice. Intranasal naloxone for rescue use should be offered to opioid-treated patients who are at increased risk for overdose (e.g., patients taking ≥50 MME/day or concurrently taking benzodiazepines, gabapentinoids, or other CNS depressants).[27] Naloxone has a short half-life and repeated dosing may be needed, especially for overdose with a long-acting or extended-release opioid agonist.

Nalmefene, which was recently returned to the market in a generic injectable formulation, has a longer duration of action than many opioid analgesics, and it could precipitate a dangerously prolonged period of withdrawal in patients dependent on opioids. Data are lacking on use of nalmefene for reversal of overdose due to fentanyl or its analogues.[28]

FULL OPIOID AGONISTS

CODEINE — Codeine is an oral opioid agonist with a long history of use as an analgesic and cough suppressant. It is a prodrug that is converted to morphine by CYP2D6. Patients who are CYP2D6 poor metabolizers or are taking a CYP2D6 inhibitor (e.g., fluoxetine, paroxetine, bupropion) may be unable to convert codeine to morphine and may not experience an analgesic effect.[21] Patients who are CYP2D6 ultra-rapid metabolizers convert codeine to higher-than-usual levels of morphine, which may result in toxicity.

The FDA has issued warnings about the use of codeine in children due to concerns about the risk of respiratory depression and death. The drug is contraindicated for use in children <12 years old for any indication and in those <18 years old after tonsillectomy or adenoidectomy. Codeine should be avoided in children 12-18 years old who are obese or have an increased risk of serious breathing problems and in breastfeeding women.[29]

FENTANYL — Fentanyl is available in parenteral, transdermal, intra-nasal, and oral transmucosal formulations. It is FDA-approved only for use in opioid-tolerant patients. Fentanyl should be started only after initial titration with a short-acting opioid.

Exposure of a fentanyl patch to an external heat source (e.g., a sauna, hot tub, or heating pad), increased exertion, or high fever could increase release of the drug and the risk of respiratory depression.[30] Deaths have occurred in children following accidental exposure to the patch. The FDA recommends disposing of the patch by folding the sticky sides together and flushing it down the toilet or by returning it to the pharmacy for safe disposal.[31]

HYDROCODONE — Hydrocodone is an oral semi-synthetic opioid that is partly metabolized by CYP2D6 to hydromorphone. Immediate-release formulations have been available for years in various fixed-dose combinations. Extended-release, single-entity hydrocodone products are available for management of severe pain; they permit higher dosing than immediate-release combination formulations.[32,33]

An oral, immediate-release, fixed-dose combination of benzhydrocodone, a prodrug of hydrocodone, and acetaminophen *(Apadaz)* is FDA-approved for short-term (<14 days) management of severe acute pain.

HYDROMORPHONE — A semi-synthetic opioid and a metabolite of hydrocodone, hydromorphone is available in parenteral, rectal, and immediate- and extended-release oral formulations.[34] In an open-label study in patients with chronic noncancer pain, once-daily hydromorphone was similar in efficacy to twice-daily oxycodone and caused less somnolence.[35] The initial dosage of hydromorphone should be reduced in patients with moderate to severe renal impairment.

LEVORPHANOL — Oral levorphanol is used for treatment of chronic pain. It has a long half-life (16-18 hours) and can accumulate with repeated dosing.

MEPERIDINE — Meperidine should only be used for short-term (24-48 hours) treatment of moderate to severe acute pain. It is shorter-acting than morphine. Meperidine has poor oral bioavailability, is highly irritating to tissues when given subcutaneously, and it can cause muscle fibrosis when given intramuscularly.

Table 2. Some Oral/Transdermal Opioid Analgesics

Drug	Some Oral/Transdermal Formulations	Usual Adult Initial Dosage[1]
Full Agonists		
Codeine – generic	15, 30, 60 mg tabs	15-60 mg q4h
Fentanyl transdermal – generic	12, 25, 37.5, 50, 62.5, 75, 87.5, 100 mcg/hr patches	See footnotes 6,7
transmucosal –		
Actiq (Teva) generic	200, 400, 600, 800, 1200, 1600 mcg transmucosal lozenges	200 mcg
Fentora (Cephalon) generic	100, 200, 400, 600, 800 mcg buccal tabs	100 mcg
Lazanda (West)	100, 400 mcg/100 mcL nasal spray	100 mcg
Subsys (West)	100, 200, 400, 600, 800, 1200, 1600 mcg sublingual spray	100 mcg

MME = oral morphine milligram equivalent

1. Dosage for patients who are opioid-naive or opioid-nontolerant (products such as fentanyl are not recommended for such patients). In general, experts recommend starting with the lowest available strength of an immediate-release opioid and titrating to effect; in opioid-naive patients, it would be reasonable to start with 5-10 mg of morphine per dose or 20-30 mg per day, or its equivalent (see MME conversion factors above). For acute pain, an immediate-release formulation of a full opioid agonist should be used as needed (i.e., not around the clock). Dosage adjustment for renal or hepatic impairment may be necessary.
2. Approximate WAC for 30 days' treatment at the lowest usual adult oral starting dosage or with the lowest available strength. WAC = wholesaler acquisition cost or manufacturer's published price to wholesalers; WAC represents a published catalogue or list price and may not represent an actual transactional price. Source: AnalySource® Monthly. November 5, 2022. Reprinted with permission by First Databank, Inc. All rights reserved. ©2022. www.fdbhealth.com/policies/drug-pricing-policy.
3. Single-agent codeine is a schedule II controlled substance; fixed-dose combinations containing acetaminophen are schedule III or V.

Comments	Cost[2]
▸ Schedule II-V[3] controlled substance	$129.40
▸ Metabolized to morphine by CYP2D6	
▸ MME conversion factor[4]: 0.15[5]	
▸ Also available in fixed-dose combinations with acetaminophen	
▸ Contraindicated in all children <12 years old and in those <18 years old post-adenoidectomy or tonsillectomy	
▸ Schedule II controlled substance	
▸ MME conversion factor[4]:	162.40
patch[8]: 2.4	
tabs/lozenges[9]: 0.13	
nasal spray[9]: 0.16	87.40[10]
sublingual spray[9]: 0.18	12.20[10]
▸ Also available parenterally	
▸ Not recommended for opioid-naive patients	68.50[10]
▸ *Actiq, Fentora, Lazanda,* and *Subsys* are indicated only for breakthrough pain in opioid-tolerant patients with cancer	46.40[10]
	127.40[10]
▸ *Actiq* may cause dental caries	
	76.60[10]

4. To convert the total daily dose of an opioid (except fentanyl: see footnotes 6 and 7) to MMEs, multiply its dose in mg/day by the conversion factor. The conversion factor is an estimate and should not be used to determine the dosage for converting patients from one opioid to another. When converting patients from one opioid to another, the new opioid is typically dosed substantially lower (25-50%) than the calculated dose in MMEs (CDC National Center for Injury Prevention and Control. Available at: http://bit.ly/3g5Uz3E. Accessed November 21, 2022).
5. MME conversion factor varies with CYP2D6 metabolizer status.
6. Starting dose determined by previous opioid dosage. Extended-release/long-acting formulations are generally not recommended for opioid-naive patients.
7. Not recommended for opioid-nontolerant patients. The recommended dosing interval is 72 hours. Some patients need to change the patch every 48 hours to achieve adequate analgesia.
8. To convert the fentanyl patch to the MME dose/day, multiply the dose in mcg/hr by the conversion factor.
9. To convert fentanyl transmucosal products to MMEs, multiply the number of micrograms in a given unit by the conversion factor.
10. Cost for a single lozenge, tablet, or spray of the lowest available strength.

Continued on next page

Table 2. Some Oral/Transdermal Opioid Analgesics (continued)		
Drug	**Some Oral/Transdermal Formulations**	**Usual Adult Initial Dosage[1]**
Full Agonists (continued)		
Hydrocodone – extended-release – generic	10, 15, 20, 30, 40, 50 mg ER caps	10 mg q12h[6,11]
Hysingla ER (Purdue)* generic	20, 30, 40, 60, 80, 100, 120 mg ER tabs	20 mg q24h[6]
Benzhydrocodone/ acetaminophen – *Apadaz* (KVK Tech) generic	4.08 mg, 6.12 mg, 8.16 mg/ 325 mg tabs	6.12 mg/325 mg q4-6h
Hydromorphone – generic *Dilaudid* (Rhodes)	2, 4, 8 mg tabs; 5 mg/5 mL PO soln	2 mg q6-8h
extended-release – generic	8, 12, 16, 32 mg ER tabs	See footnote 6
Levorphanol – generic	2, 3 mg tabs	2 mg q6-8h
Meperidine – generic	50 mg tabs; 50 mg/5 mL PO soln	50 mg q3-4h
Methadone – generic	5, 10 mg tabs; 5, 10 mg/5 mL PO soln; 10 mg/mL PO conc; 40 mg tabs for PO susp	2.5-10 mg q8-12h[6]

*FDA-approved as an abuse-deterrent formulation; ER = extended-release; MME = oral morphine milligram equivalent
11. Concurrent use of alcohol can increase peak hydrocodone concentrations and should be avoided.
12. Cost of 30 8-mg tablets.

Comments	Cost[2]
▸ Schedule II controlled substance ▸ MME conversion factor[4]: 1 ▸ Immediate-release formulations only available in fixed-dose combinations with acetaminophen, ibuprofen, homatropine, or guaifenesin	$449.30 328.00 241.10
▸ Schedule II controlled substance ▸ Prodrug of hydrocodone ▸ Only available in a fixed-dose combination with acetaminophen	31.20 31.20
▸ Schedule II controlled substance ▸ MME conversion factor[4]: 4 ▸ Also available in parenteral formulations, including a high-potency injectable, and as a suppository	17.50 279.30 218.40[12]
▸ Schedule II controlled substance ▸ MME conversion factor[4]: 11 ▸ Accumulation may occur with chronic use	3629.90
▸ Schedule II controlled substance ▸ MME conversion factor[4]: 0.1 ▸ Also available parenterally ▸ Tissue irritation occurs with parenteral use ▸ Use should be limited to ≤48 hours	447.50[13]
▸ Schedule II controlled substance ▸ MME conversion factor[4]: variable[14] ▸ Also available parenterally ▸ Accumulation may occur with chronic use	$9.70

13. Cost for 2 days' treatment.
14. The methadone conversion factor is 4 at doses of 1-20 mg/day, 8 at doses of 21-40 mg/day, 10 at doses at 41-60 mg/day, and 12 at doses of 61-80 mg/day.

Continued on next page

Table 2. Some Oral/Transdermal Opioid Analgesics (continued)		
Drug	**Some Oral/Transdermal Formulations**	**Usual Adult Initial Dosage[1]**
Full Agonists (continued)		
Morphine – generic	15, 30 mg tabs; 10, 20, 100 mg/5 mL PO soln	10 mg q4h
extended-release – generic		
MS Contin (Rhodes)	15, 30, 60, 100, 200 mg ER tabs	15-30 mg q8-12h[6]
generic	10, 20, 30, 50, 60, 80, 100 mg ER caps	30 mg q24h[6]
multiphase – generic	30, 45, 60, 75, 90, 120 mg ER caps	30 mg q24h[6]
Oxycodone – generic	5 mg caps; 5, 10, 15, 20, 30 mg tabs; 5, 100 mg/5 mL PO soln	5-15 mg q4-6h
Oxaydo (Egalet)	5, 7.5 mg tabs	
Roxybond (Daiichi Sankyo)*	5, 15, 30 mg tabs	
extended-release –		10 mg q12h[6]
OxyContin (Purdue)*	10, 15, 20, 30, 40, 60, 80 mg ER tabs	
generic		9 mg q12h[6]
Xtampza ER (Collegium)*	9, 13.5, 18, 27, 36 mg ER caps	
Oxymorphone – generic	5, 10 mg tabs	5-15 mg q4-6h
extended-release – generic	5, 7.5, 10, 15, 20, 30, 40 mg ER tabs	5 mg q12h[6]
Full Agonist/Reuptake Inhibitors		
Tapentadol –		
Nucynta (Collegium)	50, 75, 100 mg tabs	50-100 mg q4-6h
extended-release –	50, 100, 150, 200, 250 mg ER tabs	50 mg bid[6]
Nucynta ER		

*FDA-approved as an abuse-deterrent formulation; ER = extended-release; MME = oral morphine milligram equivalent

Comments	Cost[2]
► Schedule II controlled substance	$62.60[15]
► Also available for parenteral use and as a suppository	
► Taking ER caps with alcohol can result in rapid release of morphine	31.70
► Maximum dose of multiphase ER caps is 1600 mg because of renal toxicity of fumaric acid in the beads (chewing or crushing the beads can be fatal)	252.60
	136.50
	137.50
► Schedule II controlled substance	30.20
► MME conversion factor[4]: 1.5	
► Also available in fixed-dose combinations with acetaminophen, aspirin, or ibuprofen	1169.70
	1311.60
	279.50
	198.40
	355.00
► Schedule II controlled substance	112.80
► MME conversion factor[4]: 3	218.50
► Also available parenterally	
► Schedule II controlled substance	
► MME conversion factor[4]: 0.4	1060.30
► Fewer GI adverse effects, but similar CNS effects compared to some other opioid agonists	570.90

15. Cost of 15-mg tabs.

Continued on next page

Table 2. Some Oral/Transdermal Opioid Analgesics (continued)		
Drug	**Some Oral/Transdermal Formulations**	**Usual Adult Initial Dosage[1]**
Full Agonist/Reuptake Inhibitors (continued)		
Tramadol – generic	50 mg tabs	50-100 mg q4-6h
oral solution – generic	25 mg/5 mL oral soln	
extended-release –		
generic	100, 200, 300 mg ER tabs	
multiphase – generic	100, 200, 300 mg ER tabs	100 mg once/day[6]
biphasic – generic	100, 200, 300 mg ER caps[16]	
ConZip (Vertical)		

ER = extended-release; MME = oral morphine milligram equivalent
16. Mixture of immediate-release (IR) and extended-release (ER) tramadol: 100 mg contains 25 mg IR and 75 mg ER, 200 mg contains 50 mg IR and 150 mg ER, 300 mg contains 50 mg IR and 250 mg ER.

Repeated doses of meperidine can lead to accumulation of normeperidine, a toxic metabolite with a 15- to 30-hour half-life. Normeperidine can cause dysphoria, irritability, tremor, myoclonus, and, occasionally, seizures, particularly with postoperative patient-controlled analgesia, or in elderly patients or those with impaired renal function.

METHADONE — Methadone is available orally and parenterally for treatment of chronic pain and orally for maintenance treatment of opioid use disorder.[9] In one study, methadone was similar in efficacy to long-acting morphine for first-line treatment of cancer pain.[36]

The plasma half-life of methadone is variable and does not correlate with the duration of analgesia; close monitoring is required during the titration period because repeated doses can lead to accumulation, CNS depression,

Comments	Cost[2]
▸ Schedule IV controlled substance	$5.60
▸ Metabolized by CYP2D6 to a more active metabolite	2378.40
▸ MME conversion factor[4]: 0.1[5]	
▸ 50 mg equivalent to codeine 60 mg; 100 mg comparable	75.60
to aspirin 650 mg plus codeine 60 mg	45.50
▸ Also available in fixed-dose combinations with acetaminophen	229.60
or celecoxib	369.20
▸ Contraindicated in all children <12 years old and in those <18 years old post-adenoidectomy or tonsillectomy	
▸ Starting with 25 mg/day and slowly titrating to usual dose over a few weeks may improve tolerability	
▸ Maximum dose is 400 mg/day for immediate-release formulations and 300 mg/day for ER formulations	

and death. In comparison to other opioids, use of methadone for pain relief has been associated with a higher risk of death from overdose.[37]

In addition to being a mu-agonist, methadone is also an NMDA (*N*-methyl-D-aspartate) receptor antagonist. NMDA receptor antagonism can be helpful when other opioids are ineffective, particularly in treating neuropathic pain. Switching from another opioid agonist to methadone should be done cautiously by an experienced clinician; the equianalgesic dose of methadone is not well established in opioid-tolerant patients.

Methadone has no active metabolites, which may be advantageous in patients with renal impairment. Dose-related QT-interval prolongation, torsades de pointes, and death have been reported.[38]

MORPHINE — Morphine is available in parenteral, rectal, and immediate- and extended-release oral formulations. After oral administration, morphine undergoes extensive first-pass metabolism, resulting in a bioavailability of about 35%. It commonly causes nausea, vomiting, and constipation. Morphine should be used with caution in patients with severe renal impairment because accumulation of its metabolites can occur. Increased concentrations of morphine-3-glucuronide, a neurotoxic metabolite, can cause agitation, confusion, delirium, and other adverse effects. Morphine-6-glucuronide maintains activity as an opioid agonist and could increase toxicity in persons with renal impairment.

OLICERIDINE – An IV opioid, oliceridine *(Olinvyk)* couples the mu-opioid receptor preferentially to G proteins, reducing activation of the beta-arrestin pathway, which theoretically could decrease the risk of opioid adverse effects. In two 48-hour trials, it was not superior to morphine in relieving moderate to severe acute postoperative pain. Oliceridine appears to cause less GI toxicity than morphine, but its maximum daily dose is limited by a risk of QT-interval prolongation, and it is expensive.[39]

OXYCODONE — Oxycodone, a semi-synthetic opioid, is only available in oral formulations in the US. It is frequently used in combination with acetaminophen for treatment of acute pain. A long-acting formulation is commonly used for treatment of chronic pain.

OXYMORPHONE — A metabolite of oxycodone, oxymorphone is available in parenteral and immediate- and extended-release oral formulations.[40] *Opana ER*, an oral extended-release formulation of oxymorphone, was removed from the market because of a high risk of abuse[41]; generic formulations of oral extended-release oxymorphone remain available.

ABUSE-DETERRENT OPIOIDS — Several full-agonist opioids are available in "abuse-deterrent" formulations (see Table 2). These formulations have one or more properties that make their intentional nontherapeutic use more difficult, less attractive, or less rewarding. No studies comparing the relative safety of these products are available. Whether using them actually reduces overall opioid abuse remains to be established. No opioid formulation prevents consumption of a large number of intact dosage units, the most common method of abuse.[42-44]

FULL AGONIST/REUPTAKE INHIBITORS

TAPENTADOL — Tapentadol is an opioid agonist and a norepinephrine reuptake inhibitor. It is available in immediate- and extended-release oral formulations.[45] The extended-release formulation appears to provide analgesic efficacy similar to that of extended-release oxycodone with fewer GI adverse effects.[46] Tapentadol is contraindicated for use with or within 14 days of taking an MAO inhibitor.

TRAMADOL — Tramadol is an oral, centrally-acting opioid agonist that inhibits reuptake of norepinephrine and serotonin. It is metabolized by CYP2D6 to a metabolite that is 2-4 times more active than the parent drug; CYP2D6 poor metabolizers and patients taking a CYP2D6 inhibitor may not experience an analgesic effect.[21] Tramadol is available alone and in combination with acetaminophen and with celecoxib *(Seglentis)*.[47] The combination of tramadol and acetaminophen for treatment of chronic pain is comparable in efficacy to that of oxycodone plus acetaminophen. The need for slow dose titration to decrease nausea and improve tolerability when initiating tramadol limits its use for treatment of acute pain. Tramadol may be effective for treatment of neuropathic pain, but the supporting evidence is weak.[48]

Seizures have been reported with tramadol; patients with a history of seizures and those who are also taking a tricyclic antidepressant, an SSRI, an MAO inhibitor, other opioids, or an antipsychotic drug may be at increased risk. Administration of naloxone for an overdose of tramadol may increase seizure risk. Concentrations of the active metabolite of tramadol may be higher in CYP2D6 ultra-rapid metabolizers, resulting in a higher incidence of adverse effects. Concurrent use of tramadol with drugs that inhibit CYP2D6 or 3A4 can increase tramadol levels and seizure risk.[21]

Hyponatremia has been reported with use of tramadol, particularly during the first week of treatment in women ≥65 years old. Severe hypoglycemia has also been reported with use of the drug, particularly in patients with risk factors such as diabetes.[49] Serotonin syndrome can occur with use of tramadol.

The FDA has issued warnings about cases of life-threatening respiratory depression and death that occurred in children who received tramadol. The drug is contraindicated for use in children <12 years old for any indication and in those <18 years old after tonsillectomy or adenoidectomy. Use of tramadol should be avoided in children 12-18 years old who are obese or have an increased risk of serious breathing problems and in breastfeeding women.[29]

A PARTIAL AGONIST

The partial opioid agonist buprenorphine, which is commonly used for treatment of opioid use disorder,[9] is also available in oral transmucosal *(Belbuca)* and parenteral formulations *(Buprenex*, and generics), and in a transdermal patch *(Butrans)* for treatment of pain. In some studies, oral or transdermal buprenorphine was effective in reducing pain in patients with chronic back pain.[50,51] Because of the low maximum dose of the patch (20 mcg/hr), it is not useful for treatment of severe cancer pain. Patients maintained on transdermal buprenorphine may require higher-than-normal doses of full opioid agonists during and for up to 48 hours following discontinuation of the patch.

Buprenorphine has a ceiling on its respiratory depressant effect and a lower abuse potential than full opioid agonists. Nausea, headache, dizziness, and somnolence are common adverse effects, and it can precipitate withdrawal in persons taking full opioid agonists.

MIXED AGONIST/ANTAGONISTS

The mixed opioid agonist/antagonists pentazocine, butorphanol, and nalbuphine all have a ceiling on their analgesic effects and can precipitate withdrawal symptoms in patients physically dependent on full opioid agonists. These drugs are less likely than full agonists to cause physical dependence, but none is entirely free of dependence liability.

1. D Dowell et al. CDC clinical practice guideline for prescribing opioids for pain–United States, 2022. MMWR Recomm Rep 2022; 71:1.
2. Nonopioid drugs for pain. Med Lett Drugs Ther 2022; 64:33.
3. AK Chang et al. Effect of a single dose of oral opioid and nonopioid analgesics on acute extremity pain in the emergency department: a randomized clinical trial. JAMA 2017; 318:1661.
4. R Chou et al. Treatments for acute pain: a systematic review [Internet]. Comparative effectiveness review #240. Rockville (MD): Agency for Healthcare Research and Quality (US); December 2020. Report No.: 20(21)-EHC006. Available at: http://bit.ly/3UCZzvR. Accessed November 21, 2022.
5. CJ Derry et al. Caffeine as an analgesic adjuvant for acute pain in adults. Cochrane Database Syst Rev 2014; 2014(12):CD009281.
6. M Miller et al. Prescription opioid duration of action and the risk of unintentional overdose among patients receiving opioid therapy. JAMA Intern Med 2015; 175:608.
7. RA Deyo et al. Association between initial opioid prescribing patterns and subsequent long-term use among opioid-naïve patients: a statewide retrospective cohort study. J Gen Intern Med 2017; 32:21.
8. A Shah et al. Characteristics of initial prescription episodes and likelihood of long-term opioid use - United States, 2006-2015. MMWR Morb Mortal Wkly Rep 2017; 66:265.
9. Drugs for opioid use disorder. Med Lett Drugs Ther 2017; 59:89.
10. R Chou et al. The effectiveness and risks of long-term opioid therapy for chronic pain: a systematic review for a National Institutes of Health Pathways of Prevention Workshop. Ann Intern Med 2015; 162:276.
11. DR Veiga et al. Effectiveness of opioids for chronic noncancer pain: a two-year multicenter, prospective cohort study with propensity score matching. J Pain 2019; 20:706.
12. EE Krebs et al. Effect of opioid vs nonopioid medications on pain-related function in patients with chronic back pain or hip or knee osteoarthritis pain: the SPACE randomized clinical trial. JAMA 2018; 319:872.
13. Methylnaltrexone (Relistor) for opioid-induced constipation. Med Lett Drugs Ther 2008; 50:63.
14. Naloxegol (Movantik) for opioid-induced constipation. Med Lett Drugs Ther 2015; 57:135.
15. Naldemedine (Symproic) for opioid-induced constipation. Med Lett Drugs Ther 2017; 59:196.

16. Lubiprostone (Amitiza) for opioid-induced constipation. Med Lett Drugs Ther 2013; 55:47.

17. M Lee et al. A comprehensive review of opioid-induced hyperalgesia. Pain Physician 2011; 14:145.

18. MJ Brennan. The effect of opioid therapy on endocrine function. Am J Med 2013; 126:S12.

19. FDA Drug Safety Communication: FDA warns about several safety issues with opioid pain medicines; requires label changes. March 22, 2016. Available at: http://bit.ly/3AiIT4w. Accessed November 21, 2022.

20. FDA Drug Safety Communication: FDA warns about serious risks and death when combining opioid pain or cough medicines with benzodiazepines; requires its strongest warning. August 31, 2016. Available at: http://bit.ly/3UInBW8. Accessed November 21, 2022.

21. Inhibitors and inducers of CYP enzymes, P-glycoprotein, and other transporters. Med Lett Drugs Ther 2021 October 20 (epub). Available at www.medicalletter.org/downloads/CYP_PGP_Tables.pdf. Accessed November 21, 2022.

22. Drug interactions: opioids and oral $P2Y_{12}$ platelet inhibitors. Med Lett Drugs Ther 2019; 61:31.

23. RHM Furtado et al. Morphine and cardiovascular outcomes among patients with non-ST-segment elevation acute coronary syndromes undergoing coronary angiography. J Am Coll Cardiol 2020; 75:289.

24. VE Whiteman et al. Maternal opioid drug use during pregnancy and its impact on perinatal morbidity, mortality, and the costs of medical care in the United States. J Pregnancy 2014; 2014:906723.

25. RE Azuine et al. Prenatal risk factors and perinatal and postnatal outcomes associated with maternal opioid exposure in an urban, low-income, multiethnic US population. JAMA Netw Open 2019; 2:e196405.

26. Substance Abuse and Mental Health Services Administration. Clinical guidance for treating pregnant and parenting women with opioid use disorder and their infants. HHS Publication No. (SMA) 18-5054. Rockville, MD: 2018. Available at: http://bit.ly/3OaIZkr. Accessed November 21, 2022.

27. HHS. Naloxone: the opioid reversal drug that saves lives. Available at: https://bit.ly/3k68NiV. Accessed November 21, 2022.

28. Nalmefene returns for reversal of opioid overdose. Med Lett Drugs Ther 2022; 64:141.

29. FDA warns against use of codeine and tramadol in children and breastfeeding women. Med Lett Drugs Ther 2017; 59:86.

30. In brief: Heat and transdermal fentanyl. Med Lett Drugs Ther 2009; 51:64.

31. FDA Drug Safety Communication: FDA requiring color changes to Duragesic (fentanyl) pain patches to aid safety—emphasizing that accidental exposure to used patches can cause death. September 23, 2013. Available at: http://bit.ly/3GkUxzO. Accessed November 21, 2022.

32. Extended-release hydrocodone (Zohydro ER) for pain. Med Lett Drugs Ther 2014; 56:45.

33. Extended-release hydrocodone (Hysingla ER) for pain. Med Lett Drugs Ther 2015; 57:71.

34. Extended-release hydromorphone (Exalgo) for pain. Med Lett Drugs Ther 2011; 53:62.

35. H Binsfeld et al. A randomized study to demonstrate noninferiority of once-daily OROS hydromorphone with twice-daily sustained-release oxycodone for moderate to severe chronic noncancer pain. Pain Pract 2010; 10:404.

36. E Bruera et al. Methadone versus morphine as a first-line strong opioid for cancer pain: a randomized, double-blind study. J Clin Oncol 2004; 22:185.

37. M Faul et al. Methadone prescribing and overdose and the association with Medicaid preferred drug list policies — United States, 2007–2014. MMWR Morb Mortal Wkly Rep 2017; 66:320.

38. MJ Krantz et al. QTc interval screening in methadone treatment. Ann Intern Med 2009; 150:387.

39. Oliceridine (Olinvyk) - a new opioid for severe pain. Med Lett Drugs Ther 2021; 63:37.

40. Oral oxymorphone (Opana). Med Lett Drugs Ther 2007; 49:3.

41. FDA. Oxymorphone (marketed as Opana ER) information. February 6, 2018. Available at: https://bit.ly/3Gv2UJa. Accessed: November 21, 2022.

42. Abuse-deterrent opioid formulations. Med Lett Drugs Ther 2015; 57:119.

43. Arymo ER – a new abuse-deterrent morphine formulation. Med Lett Drugs Ther 2017; 59:68.

44. A new abuse-deterrent opioid – Xtampza ER. Med Lett Drugs Ther 2016; 58:77.

45. Tapentadol (Nucynta) – a new analgesic. Med Lett Drugs Ther 2009; 51:61.

46. M Afilalo and B Morlion. Efficacy of tapentadol ER for managing moderate to severe chronic pain. Pain Physician 2013; 16:27.

47. Tramadol/celecoxib (Seglentis) for pain. Med Lett Drugs Ther 2022; 64:58.

48. RM Duehmke et al. Tramadol for neuropathic pain in adults. Cochrane Database Syst Rev 2017; 6:CD003726.

49. JP Fournier et al. Tramadol use and the risk of hospitalization for hypoglycemia in patients with noncancer pain. JAMA Intern Med 2015; 175:186.

50. Transdermal buprenorphine (Butrans) for chronic pain. Med Lett Drugs Ther 2011; 53:31.

51. Buprenorphine buccal film (Belbuca) for chronic pain. Med Lett Drugs Ther 2016; 58:47.

DRUGS FOR
Sexually Transmitted Infections

Original publication date – June 2022

This article includes recommendations for management of most sexually transmitted infections (STIs) other than HIV and viral hepatitis. Some of the indications and dosages recommended here have not been approved by the FDA (see Table 1).

PARTNER TREATMENT — Management of all STIs should include evaluation of recent sex partners of infected persons. If possible, partners should be examined and tested for STIs, but in most cases partner treatment of bacterial STIs and trichomoniasis should be started regardless of symptoms and without waiting for laboratory test results.

An alternative approach is to treat sex partners without direct examination or testing, by either writing a prescription or giving the medication for the partner to the index patient, a practice called expedited partner therapy (EPT). EPT is legally permissible or potentially allowable in all 50 states in the US.[1]

CHLAMYDIA — Chlamydial infection is the most frequently reported bacterial infectious disease in the US.[2] Asymptomatic infection is common. The regimen of choice for treatment of oropharyngeal, urogenital, and rectal *Chlamydia trachomatis* infections is 7 days of oral doxycycline. Oral levofloxacin is an effective alternative. A single

Table 1. Drugs of Choice for Some STIs[1]

Type or Stage	Regimen(s) of Choice
Chlamydial Infection	
Oropharyngeal, urogenital, or rectal (not LGV)	Doxycycline 100 mg PO bid x 7 days[2,3]
Infection in pregnancy	Azithromycin 1 g PO once
Neonatal ophthalmia or pneumonia	Erythromycin 12.5 mg/kg PO qid x 14 days[6,7]
Lymphogranuloma venereum (LGV)	Doxycycline 100 mg PO bid x 21days[2]
Nongonococcal urethritis/cervicitis[10]	Doxycycline 100 mg PO bid x 7 days[2,11]
Gonorrhea	
Urogenital or rectal	Ceftriaxone 500 mg (<150 kg) or 1 g (≥150 kg) IM once[12]
Pharyngeal	Ceftriaxone 500 mg (<150 kg) or 1 g (≥150 kg) IM once[12,15]
Conjunctivitis	Ceftriaxone 1 g IM once[17]
Arthritis/arthritis-dermatitis	Ceftriaxone 1 g IM/IV q24h[12,18]
Meningitis/endocarditis	Ceftriaxone 1-2 g IV q24h x 10-14 days (meningitis) or >4 weeks (endocarditis)[12]
Infection in pregnancy	Ceftriaxone 500 mg (<150 kg) or 1 g (≥150 kg) IM once[19]
Neonatal ophthalmia	Ceftriaxone 25-50 mg/kg IV or IM once (max 250 mg)

1. Adapted from KA Workowski et al. MMWR Recomm Rep 2021; 70:1.
2. Not recommended for use during pregnancy or in breastfeeding women.
3. Delayed-release doxycycline *(Doryx)* 200 mg once daily for 7 days is as effective as twice-daily doxycycline, with less GI toxicity, but it costs more.
4. A single dose of oral azithromycin is less effective than doxycycline for rectal chlamydial infection. Because rectal coinfection is common in women with urogenital *Chlamydia trachomatis* infection, azithromycin is no longer recommended for routine treatment of uncomplicated chlamydial infection; it remains an alternative when compliance is a concern.
5. Fluoroquinolones are generally not recommended for patients <18 years old or in pregnant or breastfeeding women.
6. Erythromycin base or ethylsuccinate. Effectiveness of erythromycin for chlamydial pneumonia and neonatal ophthalmia is about 80%; a second course may be needed.
7. Use of oral erythromycin and azithromycin in infants <6 weeks old has been associated with hypertropic pyloric stenosis.
8. Alternative regimen for chlamydial pneumonia.
9. Data are lacking; test of cure 4 weeks after completion of therapy can be considered.

Alternatives

Azithromycin 1 g PO once[4]
Levofloxacin 500 mg PO once/day x 7 days[5]

Amoxicillin 500 mg PO tid x 7 days

Azithromycin 20 mg/kg PO once/day x 3 days[7,8]

Azithromycin 1 g PO once/day x 21 days[9]
Erythromycin base 500 mg PO qid x 21 days

Azithromycin 1 g PO once[11]

Cefixime 800 mg PO once[12,13]
Gentamicin 240 mg IM once[2] plus azithromycin 2 g PO once[14]

See footnote 16

Cefotaxime or ceftizoxime 1 g IV q8 h[12,18]

See footnote 16

Cefotaxime 100 mg/kg IV or IM once[13]

---

10. In women with cervicitis, those at increased risk of gonorrhea infection should also be treated empirically for gonorrhea.
11. Some experts add a single 2-g dose of oral tinidazole or metronidazole 400 mg once/day to also treat trichomoniasis. For cases of persistent or recurrent NGU, oral doxycycline 100 mg bid for 7 days, followed by moxifloxacin 400 mg once/day for 7 days is recommended if infection with *Mycoplasma genitalium* is suspected.
12. If chlamydial infection has not been excluded, doxycycline 100 mg PO bid for 7 days should be added.
13. Only when treatment with ceftriaxone is not possible.
14. If allergic to cephalosporins.
15. Test of cure 7-14 days after initial treatment is recommended.
16. Consultation with an ID specialist is recommended for patients with a cephalosporin allergy.
17. One-time lavage of the infected eye with saline solution can be considered.
18. Oral treatment can be considered 24-48 hours after clinical improvement for a total treatment course >7 days.
19. If chlamydial infection has not been excluded, a single dose of oral azithromycin should be added.

Continued on next page

Drugs for Sexually Transmitted Infections

Table 1. Drugs of Choice for Some STIs[1] (continued)	
Type or Stage	**Regimen(s) of Choice**
Epididymitis (acute)	
	Ceftriaxone 500 mg (<150 kg) or 1 g (≥150 kg) IM once plus doxycycline 100 mg PO bid x 10 days[20]
Proctitis (acute)	
	Ceftriaxone 500 mg (<150 kg) or 1 g (≥150 kg) IM once plus doxycycline 100 mg PO bid x 7 days[2,21]
Trichomoniasis	
	Metronidazole 500 mg PO bid x 7 days (women) or 2 g PO once (men)[22]
Pelvic Inflammatory Disease	
Parenteral	Ceftriaxone 1g IV q24h[23] plus doxycycline 100 mg PO or IV q12h[2] plus metronidazole 500 mg PO or IV q12h[24] Cefotetan 2 g IV q12h or cefoxitin 2 g IV q6h[23] plus doxycycline 100 mg PO bid or IV[2,24]
IM/Oral	Ceftriaxone 500 mg (<150 kg) or 1 g (≥150 kg) IM once plus doxycycline 100 mg PO bid[2] plus metronidazole 500 mg bid x 14 days Cefoxitin 2 g IM once plus probenecid 1 g PO once plus doxycycline 100 mg PO bid[2] plus metronidazole 500 mg PO bid x 14 days

20. For treatment of acute epididymitis most likely caused by chlamydia or gonorrhea. Men at risk for chlamydia or gonorrhea and infection with enteric organisms (history of insertive anal intercourse) should receive a single 500-mg dose (1 g for person weighing ≥150 kg) of ceftriaxone IM plus a 10-day course of levofloxacin 500 mg PO once/day. For epididymitis most likely caused by enteric organisms only, treat with levofloxacin 500 mg PO once/day for 10 days.
21. Bloody discharge or perianal or mucosal ulcers among persons with acute proctitis and rectal chlamydia (NAAT) should be offered presumptive treatment for lymphogranuloma venereum with doxycycline 100 mg PO bid for 3 weeks.

Alternatives

Tinidazole 2 g PO once (women and men)[2]

Ampicillin/sulbactam 3 g IV q6h[23] plus doxycycline 100 mg PO bid or IV[2,24]
Clindamycin 900 mg IV q8h plus gentamicin 2 mg/kg IV or IM once, then
   1.5 mg/kg IV q8h[25]

Levofloxacin 500 mg PO once/day plus metronidazole 500 mg PO bid x 14 days[5,26]
Moxifloxacin 400 mg PO once/day x 14 days[5,26]
Azithromycin 500 mg IV once/day x 1-2 doses, then 250 mg PO once/day
   (total 7 days) plus metronidazole 500 mg PO bid for 12-14 days[26]

---

22. A meta-analysis found a lower rate of treatment failure with the multidose regimen compared with the single-dose regimen in HIV-negative women (K Howe and PJ Kissinger. Sex Transm Dis 2017; 44:29).
23. Parenteral therapy can be stopped 24-48 hours after clinical improvement occurs, and oral doxycycline 500 mg bid and oral metronidazole 500 mg bid should be given to complete 14 days' treatment.
24. Oral administration of doxycycline and metronidazole provide similar bioavailability to IV administration.
25. Gentamicin 3-5 mg/kg once/day can be substituted.
26. Only if IV cephalosporins cannot be administered, N. gonorrhoeae infection is unlikely, and the patient can be followed.

Continued on next page

Table 1. Drugs of Choice for Some STIs[1] (continued)	
Type or Stage	**Regimen(s) of Choice**
Syphilias[27]	
Primary, secondary, or early latent (<1 year)	Benzathine penicillin G 2.4 MU IM once
Late latent, latent of unknown duration, or tertiary	Benzathine penicillin G 2.4 MU IM once wkly x 3 wks
Neurosyphilis, ocular syphilis, or otosyphilis	Aqueous crystalline penicillin G 3-4 MU IV q4h or 18-24 MU continuous IV infusion x 10-14 days
Genital Herpes	
First episode	Acyclovir 400 mg PO tid x 7-10 days[30] Famciclovir 250 mg PO tid x 7-10 days[30] Valacyclovir 1 g PO bid x 7-10 days[30]
Episodic treatment[31,32]	Acyclovir 800 mg PO bid x 5 days or 800 mg tid x 2 days Famciclovir 1 g PO bid x 1 day or 125 mg PO bid x 5 days or 500 mg once, then 250 mg bid x 2 days Valacyclovir 500 mg PO bid x 3 days or 1 g PO once/day x 5 days
Suppression[33-35]	Acyclovir 400 mg PO bid Valacyclovir 500 mg-1 g PO once/day[36] Famciclovir 250 mg PO bid

MU = million units
27. Syphilis in pregnant women should be treated with penicillin in doses appropriate to the stage of the disease. If allergic to penicillin, skin tests, desensitization, and treatment with penicillin are recommended.
28. Efficacy not established; for use only when patient is allergic to penicillin. Adherence must be ensured.
29. Limited data indicate that ceftriaxone 1–2 g daily either IM or IV for 10–14 days can be used as an alternative treatment for neurosyphilis.
30. Treatment can be extended if healing is incomplete after 10 days of treatment.
31. Most effective if started within 1 day of lesion onset.
32. For episodic treatment in patients with HIV: valacyclovir 1 g bid, famciclovir 500 mg bid, or acyclovir 400 mg tid for 5-10 days.

Alternatives

Doxycycline 100 mg PO bid x 14 days[2,28]
Tetracycline 500 mg PO qid x 14 days[2,28]
Ceftriaxone 1 g IV or IM once/day x 10 days[28]

Doxycycline 100 mg PO bid x 4 wks[2,28]
Tetracycline 500 mg PO qid x 14 days[2,28]

Procaine penicillin G 2.4 MU IM once/day plus probenecid 500 mg PO qid x 10-14 days[29]

---

33. Discontinuing preventive treatment once/year to reassess the frequency of recurrence may be considered.
34. Suppressive therapy with acyclovir or valacyclovir should be offered to pregnant women with recurrent genital herpes beginning at 36 weeks to reduce the risk of recurrence at delivery and possibly the need for cesarean section.
35. For suppression in patients with HIV: acyclovir 400-800 mg bid, famcyclovir 500 mg bid, or valacyclovir 500 mg bid.
36. 500 mg once daily in patients with <10 recurrences per year and 500 mg bid or 1 g daily in patients with ≥10 recurrences per year. For patients with HIV, the dosage is 500 mg bid.

Continued on next page

Table 1. Drugs of Choice for Some STIs[1] (continued)	
Type or Stage	**Regimen(s) of Choice**
Anogenital Warts[37]	
Patient-applied	Imiquimod 3.75% once/day up to 8 weeks[2,38,39]
	Imiquimod 5% once/day 3x/wk up to 16 weeks[2,38,39]
	Podofilox 0.5% bid x 3 days, then 4 days off, repeat up to 4x[2]
	Sinecatechins 15% tid up to 16 weeks[2,38]
Pediculosis pubis[40]	
	Permethrin 1% cream rinse applied and washed off after 10 minutes[41]
	Pyrethrin with piperonyl butoxide applied and washed off after 10 minutes[41]
Scabies	
	Permethrin 5% cream applied and washed off after 8-14 hrs
	Ivermectin 200 mcg/kg PO x1, repeat in 14 days[42]
	Ivermectin 1% lotion applied and washed off after 8-14 hrs, repeat in 7 days

37. Recommendations for external anogenital warts. Provider-administered cryotherapy with liquid nitrogen can also be used for vaginal, urethral meatus, cervical, and intra-anal warts. Provider-administered cryoprobe should not be used in the vagina due to the risk of vaginal perforation. Trichloroacetic or bichloroacetic acid can be used for vaginal, cervical, and intra-anal warts.
38. May weaken latex condoms and diaphragms.
39. Imiquimod should be washed off 6-10 hours after application.
40. Pediculocides should not be used for infestations of the eyelashes. Such infestations are treated with petrolatum ointment applied 2-4x/day x 8-10 days.

dose of oral azithromycin is less effective than doxycycline for rectal *C. trachomatis* infection.[3,4] Azithromycin is no longer recommended for routine treatment of uncomplicated chlamydial infection because rectal coinfection is common in women with urogenital *C. trachomatis* infection. Erythromycin is no longer recommended for treatment of

Alternatives

Ivermectin 250 mcg/kg PO x 1, repeat in 7-14 days[42]
Malathion 0.5% lotion applied and washed off after 8-12 hrs[43]

Lindane 1% lotion or cream applied and washed off after 8 hrs[44]

---

41. Permethrin and pyrethrin are pediculocidal; retreatment in 7-10 days may be needed to eradicate the infestation. Some lice are resistant to pyrethrins and permethrin.
42. Ivermectin is pediculocidal, but not ovicidal; more than one dose is generally necessary to eradicate the infestation. Safety of ivermectin in pregnant women remains to be established; animal studies have shown adverse effects on the fetus. Taking ivermectin with a meal increases its bioavailability.
43. Can be used when treatment failure due to resistance is thought to have occurred. Odor and long duration of application may be difficult to tolerate.
44. For patients ≥10 years old.

chlamydial infection because GI adverse effects are common and can lead to poor adherence and treatment failure.

Pregnancy – A single dose of oral azithromycin is recommended for treatment of chlamydial infection in pregnant women.[2] Amoxicillin is a less effective alternative. Fluoroquinolones and tetracyclines are not recommended during pregnancy.

Neonates of women with untreated cervical *C. trachomatis* infection are at risk for conjunctivitis and pneumonia. Prenatal screening and treatment of pregnant women is the most effective way to prevent perinatal chlamydial infection.[5] Ophthalmic antibiotics used for prophylaxis of neonatal gonococcal ophthalmia do not prevent ocular chlamydial infection in the newborn.

Lymphogranuloma Venereum – In the US, infections with *C. trachomatis* serovars L1-L3 that cause lymphogranuloma venereum (LGV) present primarily as proctocolitis, typically in patients with rectal exposure. Patients who present with symptoms consistent with LGV (proctocolitis or genital ulcer with lymphadenopathy) should be offered presumptive treatment.[2,6] A 3-week course of oral doxycycline is recommended for treatment of LGV; oral azithromycin or erythromycin are alternatives. A shorter course of oral doxycycline (7-14 days) may be effective, but randomized controlled trials are needed.[7]

Follow-Up – Test-of-cure is generally not needed for nonpregnant patients who are treated for chlamydia with a recommended or alternative regimen; pregnant women should be tested 4 weeks after treatment is completed. All patients should be tested for reinfection 3 months after completing treatment.[2]

Partner Treatment – Sex partners should be offered treatment for chlamydia. EPT is an alternative to in-person screening, but men who have sex with men (MSM) may not be optimal candidates for EPT because they have a high risk for coexisting infections, especially undiagnosed HIV, and data on the effectiveness of EPT in reducing persistent or recurrent chlamydia in this population are limited. Asymptomatic partners of persons with LGV should be presumptively treated with a 7-day course of doxycycline.

NONGONOCOCCAL URETHRITIS AND CERVICITIS — No pathogen can be identified in 40-50% of **non-gonococcal urethritis (NGU)** cases in the US. Less than 50% of infections are caused by *C. trachomatis* and *Mycoplasma genitalium* is responsible for 15-25% of cases.[2] Other pathogens include *Trichomonas vaginalis*, *Haemophilus* species, herpes simplex virus (HSV), and adenovirus. Data on the role of *Ureaplasma* species in NGU are inconsistent.[8] Enteric organisms can cause NGU following insertive anal intercourse.

Presumptive treatment should be started at the time of diagnosis. First-line treatment of **NGU**, including chlamydial urethral and rectal infections, is a 7-day course of oral doxycycline; a single dose of oral azithromycin is an alternative. Levofloxacin is no longer recommended for treatment of NGU. Persistent or recurrent NGU in a patient who has not been re-exposed to an untreated sex partner is most commonly caused by *M. genitalium*; if infection with *M. genitalium* is suspected, a 7-day course of oral doxycycline, followed by oral moxifloxacin for 7 days, should be used.[9] A single dose of oral metronidazole or tinidazole is recommended for men who have sex with women in areas where *T. Vaginalis* is prevalent.[2]

Oral doxycycline is also recommended for presumptive treatment of **nongonococcal cervicitis**; oral azithromycin is an alternative. Women at increased risk of gonorrhea infection, such as those <25 years old and those with a new sex partner, a sex partner with concurrent partners, or a sex partner who has an STI, should also be treated empirically for gonorrhea.[2]

GONORRHEA — The treatment of choice for uncomplicated urogenital, rectal, or pharyngeal gonorrhea (if *C. trachomatis* infection has been excluded) is a single IM injection of ceftriaxone. Coadministration of azithromycin was previously used to prevent development of ceftriaxone resistance and to treat potential chlamydial co-infection, but it is no longer recommended because resistance of *Neisseria gonorrhoeae* to azithromycin is increasing. *C. trachomatis* is present in 10-30% of patients with gonorrhea; if chlamydial infection has not been excluded, oral doxycycline for 7 days should be added to ceftriaxone.

When treatment with ceftriaxone is not possible, a single 800-mg dose of oral cefixime can be used to treat uncomplicated urogenital and rectal gonorrhea; the efficacy of the drug against pharyngeal gonorrhea is limited. Due to resistance of *N. gonorrhoeae* to cefixime, the recommended dose has been increased from 400 mg to 800 mg. In patients with uncomplicated gonorrhea who have a severe allergy to penicillin or cephalosporins, a single dose of IM gentamicin plus oral azithromycin is effective in treating urogenital or rectal gonorrhea, but data on its effectiveness for treatment of pharyngeal infection are limited.[2,10]

Resistance – Over the past several decades, *N. gonorrhoeae* has progressively developed resistance to penicillin, sulfonamides, tetracyclines, and fluoroquinolones.[11-13] Gonococci have also recently demonstrated decreased susceptibility to azithromycin, cefixime, and ceftriaxone, and treatment failures have been reported in other countries. Cephalosporin resistance sufficient to result in treatment failure with the recommended regimens remains rare in the US.[2,14]

Pregnancy – Pregnant women with gonorrhea should be treated with a single dose of IM ceftriaxone; if chlamydial infection has not been excluded, a single dose of oral azithromycin should be added.

Neonatal Ocular Prophylaxis – Prenatal screening and treatment of pregnant women is the most effective way to prevent gonococcal infection in neonates. Neonatal ocular prophylaxis is required by law in most states in the US; it is no longer standard practice in Canada, where enhanced prenatal screening has been implemented. A one-time instillation of erythromycin 0.5% ophthalmic ointment in both eyes is recommended for all newborn infants, even though data on the efficacy of erythromycin ocular prophylaxis are lacking. An infant born to a mother with untreated gonorrhea should receive a single dose of IM ceftriaxone.

Follow-Up – Test-of-cure is generally not needed for patients who are treated for uncomplicated urogenital or rectal gonorrhea with a recommended or alternative regimen; it is recommended 7-14 days after treatment in patients with pharyngeal gonorrhea. Because the risk of reinfection is high, rescreening is recommended 3 months after completing treatment for all patients with gonococcal infection.[2]

Partner Treatment – Sex partners of patients with gonorrhea should be tested and presumptively treated for gonorrhea, ideally with ceftriaxone. If the partner's access to prompt clinical evaluation and treatment is limited, EPT with a single 800-mg dose of oral cefixime can be considered; doxycycline should be added for 7 days if chlamydial co-infection has not been excluded.[15,16] MSM may not be optimal candidates for EPT because they have a high risk for coexisting infections, especially undiagnosed HIV, and data on the effectiveness of EPT in reducing persistent or recurrent chlamydia in this population are limited.

EPIDIDYMITIS — For acute epididymitis in sexually active men, which is most frequently caused by *C. trachomatis or N. gonorrhoeae,* empiric treatment with a single dose of IM ceftriaxone plus oral doxycycline for 10 days is recommended. Acute epididymitis caused by enteric organisms can occur in men who practice insertive anal intercourse; a single-dose of IM ceftriaxone plus oral levofloxacin for 10 days is recommended for such patients. Older men and those who have had urinary tract instrumentation, surgery, or obstruction, or are immunosuppressed may also have epididymitis due to enteric organisms; they should be treated with oral levofloxacin for 10 days.

PROCTITIS — Acute proctitis occurs predominantly in men and women who are the receptive partner during insertive anal intercourse. It is commonly caused by *N. gonorrhoeae*, *C. trachomatis* (including LGV serovars), *Treponema pallidum,* or herpes simplex virus (HSV). Syphilitic proctitis has been reported.[17] Empiric treatment with a single dose of IM ceftriaxone plus oral doxycycline for 7 days is recommended; acyclovir or valacyclovir may be added if HSV infection is suspected. If

LGV is suspected, doxycycline treatment should be continued for a total of 3 weeks. Syphilitic proctitis should be treated with a single IM dose of benzathine penicillin G or oral doxycycline for 2 weeks.

TRICHOMONIASIS — Treatment with oral metronidazole for 7 days is recommended for all women with trichomoniasis.[18,19] A single oral dose of tinidazole is an alternative; it may be less likely than metronidazole to cause GI adverse effects, but it is more expensive. Tinidazole is often effective against metronidazole-resistant *T. vaginalis*.[20] Treatment with intravaginal metronidazole gel is not recommended. No conclusive studies have documented the efficacy of any treatment regimen in men, but single-dose metronidazole or tinidazole (alternative) is recommended. The CDC guidelines state that patients taking metronidazole do not need to abstain from drinking alcohol because the drug does not inhibit acetaldehyde dehydrogenase and therefore does not have a disulfiram-like interaction with alcohol.[2,21]

Follow-up – Reinfection is common; retesting within 3 months after treatment is recommended for all sexually active women.

Partner Treatment – Sex partners of patients with trichomoniasis should be treated with 7 days of metronidazole for women and a single dose for men.

Pregnancy – Trichomoniasis has been associated with adverse pregnancy outcomes.[22] Metronidazole appears to be safe for use during pregnancy and should be used to treat symptomatic trichomoniasis in pregnant women. The safety of tinidazole in pregnancy has not been established.

CHANCROID — Chancroid, caused by *Haemophilus ducreyi*, is currently rare in the US. A single dose of oral azithromycin or IM ceftriaxone is usually effective, but prolonged therapy or retreatment may be required in uncircumcised men and persons infected with HIV.[2,23] Treatment with oral ciprofloxacin for 3 days or erythromycin base for 7 days are alternatives, but resistance to these drugs has been reported.

Sex partners should be treated if they have had sexual contact with the infected person within 10 days of symptom onset.

PELVIC INFLAMMATORY DISEASE — *C. trachomatis* or *N. gonorrhoeae* can cause acute, nonrecurrent pelvic inflammatory disease (PID), but *Mycoplasma hominis, Haemophilus* species, and various facultative and anaerobic bacteria may also be involved as secondary pathogens. Data on the etiologic role of *M. genitalium* in PID are conflicting. Treatment regimens should include broad-spectrum antimicrobial coverage of likely pathogens, including *C. trachomatis* and *N. gonorrhoeae*. Recommended regimens include ceftriaxone plus doxycycline and metronidazole (for anaerobic coverage),[24] cefotetan plus doxycycline, or cefoxitin plus doxycycline.

Parenteral therapy is continued until 24-48 hours after clinical improvement occurs, and then oral doxycycline and oral metronidazole are used to complete 14 days of treatment. Ampicillin/sulbactam plus doxycycline or clindamycin plus gentamicin are alternative parenteral regimens. An oral alternative regimen for mild to moderate acute PID is doxycycline plus metronidazole, after a single IM dose of ceftriaxone. Levofloxacin plus metronidazole, moxifloxacin monotherapy, or azithromycin plus metronidazole can be considered in patients with a cephalosporin allergy if infection with *N. gonorrhoeae* is unlikely and the patient can be followed.[2]

SYPHILIS — Parenteral penicillin G remains the drug of choice for treating all stages of syphilis. Primary, secondary, or early latent syphilis (less than one year's duration) should be treated with a single IM injection of benzathine penicillin G. In patients with severe penicillin allergy, oral doxycycline for 14 days can be used. The emergence of azithromycin-resistant *T. pallidum* precludes the use of azithromycin for treatment of syphilis in the US. For late latent syphilis (>1 year's duration or when the duration is unknown) or tertiary syphilis (gumma or cardiovascular), treatment with 3 once-weekly doses of IM benzathine penicillin G is recommended; doxycycline for 4 weeks is an alternative when benzathine penicillin G cannot be given. All persons with tertiary syphilis should have a lumbar puncture prior to treatment, and those with late latent infection (without clinical evidence of tertiary syphilis) require neurologic, otologic, and ophthalmic examinations prior to treatment.

Pregnancy – Pregnant women with syphilis should be treated with parenteral penicillin G. For those who are allergic to penicillin, skin testing, desensitization, and treatment with penicillin G are recommended.

GENITAL HERPES — Either HSV-1 and HSV-2 can cause genital herpes, but most cases of recurrent genital herpes are caused by HSV-2. Acyclovir, famciclovir, or valacyclovir taken orally for 7-10 days can shorten the duration of pain, systemic symptoms, and viral shedding in patients with an initial genital HSV infection. Treatment can be extended if healing is incomplete after 10 days of treatment. Episodic treatment of recurrent symptomatic lesions with the same drugs can facilitate healing if treatment is started immediately upon symptom onset. Persons with HIV may need higher doses and/or longer courses of treatment. Suppressive therapy reduces symptomatic recurrences and subclinical shedding. Valacyclovir has been more effective than famciclovir for virologic suppression of recurrent genital herpes[25] and suppressive therapy with valacyclovir has been shown to reduce the frequency of HSV transmission to sex partners.[26]

Pregnancy – Pregnant women with first-episode genital herpes or recurrent herpes should be treated with oral acyclovir; the drug should be given IV for severe disease. Suppressive therapy with oral acyclovir or valacyclovir beginning at week 36 can reduce the risk of recurrence at delivery and possibly the need for cesarean section, but its efficacy in reducing the risk of neonatal HSV infection is unclear. Acyclovir is generally considered safe for use during pregnancy and while breastfeeding; valacyclovir and famciclovir appear to be safe for use during pregnancy, but data are limited.[27] A case-control study found an increased risk of gastroschisis with use of antiviral drugs immediately prior to conception and during the first trimester of pregnancy.[28]

ANOGENITAL WARTS — External anogenital warts are caused by human papillomavirus (HPV) infection, usually type 6 or 11; persistent infection with other types (16, 18, or others) cause the majority of cancers and precancers in the anogenital tract and oropharynx. No treatment has been shown to eradicate HPV or to modify the risk of cervical dysplasia or cancer, and no single treatment is uniformly effective in removing warts or preventing recurrence. Trichloroacetic acid or bichloroacetic acid, cryotherapy (with liquid nitrogen or a cryoprobe), or surgical removal remain the most widely used provider-administered treatments for external anogenital warts. Imiquimod 3.75% cream *(Zyclara)* and 5% cream *(Aldara*, and generics), podofilox 0.5% solution or gel *(Condylox*, and generics), and sinecatechins 15% ointment *(Veregen)* offer the advantage of self-application.[29] For all treatments except surgical removal, the initial response rate is 60-70%; 20-30% of responders will have a recurrence, but many recurrences will respond to a different regimen.

Pregnancy – Topical trichloroacetic acid, bichloroacetic acid, and cryotherapy can be used during pregnancy. Podofilox and sinecatechins are not recommended for use during pregnancy. Imiquimod appears to have a low risk of causing fetal abnormalities, but it should be avoided during pregnancy until more safety data become available.[2]

PEDICULOSIS PUBIS AND SCABIES — *Sarcoptes scabiei* (scabies) and *Phthirus pubis* (pubic lice) can be transmitted by intimate exposure. Topical treatment options include permethrin *(Nix*, and others) or pyrethrin with piperonyl butoxide *(Rid*, and others). Oral ivermectin *(Stromectol)* is an effective, more convenient alternative, but treatment should be repeated in 7-14 days because ivermectin does not prevent eggs from hatching.[30] Malathion 0.5% lotion is an alternative for treatment of lice, but its odor and longer duration of application have limited its use; it can be used when resistance to permethrin or pyrethrin is suspected. Lindane is an alternative for scabies, but it can cause toxicity and is only recommended if other treatments are ineffective.

Drugs for Sexually Transmitted Infections

Pregnancy – Topical permethrin and pyrethrin with piperonyl butoxide can be used in pregnant women. Oral ivermectin is not recommended; animal studies have shown adverse effects on the fetus.[31] Lindane is not recommended for pregnant or breast-feeding women.

Partner Treatment – Sex partners and those who had close personal contact with the infected person within the last month should be treated.

ADVERSE EFFECTS — Doxycycline can cause GI disturbances and photosensitivity.

Azithromycin and **erythromycin** can cause GI disturbances, headache, dizziness, vaginitis, hepatotoxicity, and QT-interval prolongation.

Fluoroquinolones can cause GI disturbances, tremors, rash, oral and vaginal *Candida* infections, eosinophilia, neutropenia, leukopenia, increased aminotransferase and serum creatinine levels, insomnia, photo-sensitivity reactions, and peripheral neuropathy. They have also been associated with hyperglycemia and severe hypoglycemia, especially in older adults and in those with diabetes. Central nervous system effects including seizures, delirium, agitation, nervousness, and disturbances in attention, memory, and orientation have occurred. Other serious adverse effects include tendinitis, tendon rupture, aortic aneurysm, exacerbation of myasthenia gravis, *Clostridioides difficile* infection, and QT-interval prolongation and torsades de pointes.

Penicillins and **cephalosporins** can cause rash, diarrhea, nausea, vomiting, allergic reactions, hemolytic anemia, neutropenia, cholestatic hepatitis, serum sickness, and seizures.

Metronidazole frequently causes a metallic taste, GI upset, and headache. Neurologic adverse effects including seizures and neuropathy have been reported, particularly at high doses and with repeat or prolonged use. The adverse effects of **tinidazole** are similar to those of metronidazole, but tinidazole may be better tolerated.

Gentamicin can cause renal impairment; the risk is higher in older patients, those with impaired renal function, and those receiving other nephrotoxic medications concomitantly. Ototoxicity, *C. difficile* infection, neuromuscular blockade, and serious hypersensitivity reactions could also occur.

Clindamycin can cause GI adverse effects and *C. difficile* infection. Skin rash is common and other allergic reactions can occur. Injection-site reactions have been reported with IV administration.

Acyclovir is generally well tolerated. GI disturbances, headache, and malaise can occur. Oral acyclovir has been rarely associated with myalgia, rash, Stevens-Johnson syndrome, neutropenia and other hematologic toxicities, tremors, lethargy, confusion, hallucinations, seizures, encephalopathy, and coma. CNS adverse effects are more likely to occur in older patients and in those with renal impairment. **Famciclovir** is generally well tolerated. Headache, nausea, and diarrhea can occur. Thrombocytopenia, confusion, hallucinations, and nephrotoxicity have been reported. Adverse effects of **valacyclovir** are similar to those with acyclovir.

DRUG INTERACTIONS — Coadministration of antacids or oral products containing calcium, magnesium, or iron can decrease absorption of oral **doxycycline** and **fluoroquinolones**; administration should be separated by several hours.

Concurrent use of **azithromycin, erythromycin,** or **fluoroquinolones** and other QT-interval-prolonging drugs can result in additive effects. Erythromycin is a moderate inhibitor of CYP3A4 and can increase serum concentrations of drugs that are metabolized by CYP3A4.

Use of **fluoroquinolones** with antihyperglycemic drugs may increase the risk of hypoglycemia. Concurrent use of fluoroquinolones and nonsteroidal anti-inflammatory drugs (NSAIDs) may lower the seizure threshold.

1. CDC. Expedited partner therapy. April 19, 2021. Available at: https://bit.ly/3t56AcK. Accessed June 7, 2022.

2. KA Workowski et al. Sexually transmitted infections treatment guidelines, 2021. MMWR Recomm Rep 2021; 70:1.
3. NHTM Dukers-Muijrers et al. Treatment effectiveness of azithromycin and doxycycline in uncomplicated rectal and vaginal *Chlamydia trachomatis* infections in women: a multicenter observational study (FemCure). Clin Infect Dis 2019; 69:1946.
4. JC Dombrowski et al. Doxycycline versus azithromycin for the treatment of rectal chlamydia in men who have sex with men: a randomized controlled trial. Clin Infect Dis 2021; 73:824.
5. S Kohlhoff and SE Cohen. Universal prenatal screening and testing and *Chlamydia trachomatis* conjunctivitis in infants. Sex Transm Dis 2021; 48:e122.
6. BP Stoner and SE Cohen. Lymphogranuloma venereum 2015: clinical presentation, diagnosis, and treatment. Clin Infect Dis 2015; 61(Suppl 8):S865.
7. R Simons et al. Observed treatment responses to short-course doxycycline therapy for rectal lymphogranuloma venereum in men who have sex with men. Sex Transm Dis 2018; 45:406.
8. LH Bachmann et al. Advances in the understanding and treatment of male urethritis. Clin Infect Dis 2015; 61(Suppl 8):S763.
9. D Getman et al. *Mycoplasma genitalium* prevalence, coinfection, and macrolide antibiotic resistance frequency in a multicenter clinical study cohort in the United States. J Clin Microbiol 2016; 54:2278.
10. In brief: New recommendations for gonococcal infection. Med Lett Drugs Ther 2021; 63:72.
11. A Derbie et al. Azithromycin resistant gonococci: a literature review. Antimicrob Resist Infect Control 2020; 9:138.
12. R Selb et al. Markedly decreasing azithromycin susceptibility of *Neisseria gonorrhoeae*, Germany, 2014 to 2021. Euro Surveill 2021;26(31):2100616.
13. KE Gieseker et al. Demographic and epidemiological characteristics associated with reduced antimicrobial susceptibility to *Neisseria gonorrhoeae* in the United States, strengthening the US response to resistant gonorrhea, 2018 to 2019. Sex Transm Dis 2021; 48(12S):S118.
14. CDC. Gonococcal isolate surveillance project (GISP) profiles, 2019. July 29, 2021. Available at: https://bit.ly/3x0jv25. Accessed June 7, 2022.
15. S St Cyr et al. Update to CDC's treatment guidelines for gonococcal infection, 2020. MMWR Morb Mortal Wkly Rep 2020; 69:1911.
16. CDC. Guidance on the use of expedited partner therapy in the treatment of gonorrhea. August 18, 2021. Available at: https://bit.ly/3Gy7154. Accessed June 7, 2022.
17. M Struyve et al. Primary syphilitic proctitis: case report and literature review. Acta Gastroenterol Belg 2018; 81:430.
18. CA Munzny et al. A comparison of single-dose versus multidose metronidazole by select clinical factors for the treatment of *Trichomonas vaginalis* in women. Sex Transm Dis 2022; 49:231.
19. PJ Kissinger et al. Diagnosis and management of *Trichomonas vaginalis*: summary of evidence reviewed for the 2021 Centers for Disease Control and Prevention sexually transmitted infections treatment guidelines. Clin Infect Dis 2022; 74(Suppl_2):S152.

20. C Alessio and P Nyirjesy. Management of resistant trichomoniasis. Curr Infect Dis Rep 2019; 21:31.
21. J-P Visapää et al. Lack of disulfiram-like reaction with metronidazole and ethanol. Ann Pharmacother 2002; 36:971.
22. OT Van Gerwen et al. Trichomoniasis and adverse birth outcomes: a systematic review and meta-analysis. BJOG 2021; 128:1907.
23. DA Lewis. Epidemiology, clinical features, diagnosis and treatment of Haemophilus ducreyi – a disappearing pathogen? Expert Rev Anti Infect Ther 2014; 12:687.
24. HC Wiesenfeld et al. A randomized controlled trial of ceftriaxone and doxycycline, with or without metronidazole, for the treatment of acute pelvic inflammatory disease. Clin Infect Dis 2021; 72:1181.
25. A Wald et al. Comparative efficacy of famciclovir and valacyclovir for suppression of recurrent genital herpes and viral shedding. Sex Transm Dis 2006; 33:529.
26. L Corey et al. Once-daily valacyclovir to reduce the risk of transmission of genital herpes. N Engl J Med 2004; 350:11.
27. B Pasternak and A Hviid. Use of acyclovir, valacyclovir, and famciclovir in the first trimester of pregnancy and the risk of birth defects. JAMA 2010; 304:859.
28. KA Ahrens et al. Antiherpetic medication use and the risk of gastroschisis: findings from the National Birth Defects Prevention Study, 1997–2007. Paediatr Perinat Epidemiol 2013; 27:340.
29. Veregen: a botanical for treatment of genital warts. Med Lett Drugs Ther 2008; 50:15.
30. Y Panahi et al. The efficacy of topical and oral ivermectin in the treatment of human scabies. Ann Parasitol 2015; 61:11.
31. IM El-Ashmawy et al. Teratogenic and cytogenetic effects of ivermectin and its interaction with P-glycoprotein inhibitor. Res Vet Sci 2011; 90:116.

DRUGS FOR
Treatment and Prevention of
Venous Thromboembolism

Original publication date – July 2022

Anticoagulants are the drugs of choice for treatment and prevention of deep venous thrombosis (DVT) and pulmonary embolism (PE), collectively referred to as venous thromboembolism (VTE). US guidelines for treatment of VTE were updated in 2020 and 2021.[1,2]

STANDARD TREATMENT — Patients with acute VTE have traditionally been **treated** initially for 5-10 days with a parenteral anticoagulant such as low-molecular-weight heparin (LMWH), fondaparinux (*Arixtra*, and generics), or unfractionated heparin (UFH) (see Table 1). Now, however, either of two direct oral anticoagulants (DOACs), apixaban *(Eliquis)* or rivaroxaban *(Xarelto)*, is often preferred for initial treatment in stable patients. After initial treatment, long-term anticoagulant therapy should be continued for at least 3 months.[3] A DOAC (apixaban, dabigatran *[Pradaxa]*, edoxaban *[Savaysa]*, or rivaroxaban) is generally preferred over the vitamin K antagonist warfarin for long-term treatment (see Table 2).

LMWH is recommended for **prevention** of VTE after major nonorthopedic surgery when postoperative prophylaxis is indicated and for hospitalized medical patients who are at increased risk of thrombosis. Rivaroxaban, apixaban, dabigatran, or aspirin is recommended for prevention of VTE after knee or hip replacement surgery.[4-7]

Recommendations

Treatment of Acute VTE

- ► Low-molecular-weight heparin (LMWH) or fondaparinux, with or without warfarin, has traditionally been used for initial treatment (5-10 days) of acute deep venous thrombosis (DVT) or pulmonary embolism (PE).
- ► Apixaban and rivaroxaban are oral alternatives that are often preferred now for initial use in stable patients.
- ► A direct oral anticoagulant (DOAC) (apixaban, dabigatran, edoxaban, or rivaroxaban) or warfarin can be used for long-term treatment. DOACs are generally preferred over warfarin.
- ► An oral factor Xa inhibitor (apixaban, edoxaban, or rivaroxaban) is recommended for treatment of VTE in patients with active cancer who are not at high risk of bleeding.
- ► Warfarin or UFH has been recommended for treatment of patients with CrCl <30 mL/min, but some clinicians now prefer apixaban.
- ► LMWH is recommended for use during pregnancy.

Duration of Anticoagulation

- ► Patients with VTE should be treated for a minimum of 3 months.
- ► Patients with unprovoked VTE and those with VTE provoked by a major persistent risk factor such as active cancer have the highest risk of recurrence; they should generally be treated for >3 months and sometimes indefinitely.

Extended Treatment

- ► After at least 3 months of anticoagulation therapy, extended treatment with low doses of apixaban or rivaroxaban can prevent symptomatic recurrences of VTE.
- ► If the anticoagulant is stopped, aspirin therapy can reduce the risk of recurrence, but aspirin is less effective than anticoagulation for secondary prevention.

Primary Prevention of VTE

- ► LMWH is recommended for prevention of VTE after major nonorthopedic surgery when postoperative prophylaxis is indicated.
- ► Apixaban, rivaroxaban, dabigatran, or aspirin is recommended for prevention of VTE after knee or hip replacement surgery.
- ► LMWH is preferred for hospitalized medical patients who are at increased risk of thrombosis.

PARENTERAL ANTICOAGULANTS

HEPARIN — Heparins act by combining with plasma antithrombin to form a complex that is more active in neutralizing thrombin and factor Xa than antithrombin alone. UFH has some disadvantages compared to LMWH: it is more likely to cause heparin-induced thrombocytopenia and has a more variable anticoagulant response that requires monitoring. However, UFH also has some advantages over LMWH: its anticoagulant effect can be rapidly and completely reversed by protamine, it is not renally eliminated and may be safer in patients with renal impairment, and it directly inhibits the contact activation pathway that is important in the formation of thrombi in stents, catheters, and extracorporeal circuits.[8,9] The shorter half-life of UFH may also be advantageous in patients who are at high risk of bleeding.

LMWH — The low-molecular-weight heparins enoxaparin (*Lovenox*, and generics) and dalteparin *(Fragmin)*, which are produced by cleaving UFH into shorter chains, inhibit factor Xa more than they inhibit thrombin. Compared to UFH, LMWH has a longer half-life, which allows use of fewer doses per day. LMWH also binds less to platelets and plasma proteins, which results in greater bioavailability and a more predictable anticoagulant response. In clinical trials comparing it with UFH, LMWH has generally been as effective and at least as safe for prevention and treatment of VTE. For initial treatment of VTE in stable patients, LMWH is generally preferred over UFH.

FONDAPARINUX — A synthetic analog of the pentasaccharide sequence of heparin, fondaparinux binds antithrombin with high affinity and indirectly inhibits factor Xa. The drug has a long half-life and requires injection only once daily. Fondaparinux appears to be as effective as UFH or LMWH for prevention and treatment of VTE, and it is much less likely to cause heparin-induced thrombocytopenia. Fondaparinux accumulates in patients with renal impairment; it is contraindicated for use in patients with CrCl <30 mL/min.

Table 1. Some Parenteral Anticoagulants for VTE[1]	
Drug	**Usual Adult Treatment Dosage[2]**
Unfractionated Heparin (UFH)	
generic	80 units/kg IV bolus, then 18 units/kg/hr IV[5]
Low-Molecular-Weight Heparins (LMWHs)	
Dalteparin – *Fragmin* (Pfizer)	200 IU/kg SC once/day[5-7]
Enoxaparin – generic *Lovenox* (Sanofi)	1 mg/kg SC bid or 1.5 mg/kg SC once/day[5,6]
Factor Xa Inhibitor	
Fondaparinux – generic *Arixtra* (Mylan)	5-10 mg SC once/day[5,6,8,9]

1. See Table 4 on pages 204-205 for FDA-approved VTE indications.
2. Initial treatment is usually continued for 5-10 days.
3. Prophylaxis is recommended for a minimum of 10-14 days and for up to 35 days after major orthopedic surgery (Y Falck-Ytter et al. Chest 2012; 141:e278S).
4. Approximate WAC for 30 days' treatment of a 70-kg patient at the lowest usual adult dosage for treatment. WAC = wholesaler acquisition cost or manufacturer's published price to wholesalers; WAC represents a published catalogue or list price and may not represent an actual transactional price. Source: AnalySource® Monthly. July 5, 2022. Reprinted with permission by First Databank, Inc. All rights reserved. ©2022. www.fdbhealth.com/policies/drug-pricing-policy.
5. If warfarin is to be used, it is generally started at the same time; the parenteral anticoagulant can be stopped after a minimum of 5 days when the INR is ≥2 for at least 24 hours (MA Smythe et al. J Thromb Thrombolysis 2016; 41:165). If dabigatran or edoxaban is to be used, it should be preceded by at least 5 days of initial treatment with a parenteral anticoagulant. Apixaban and rivaroxaban do not require pretreatment with a parenteral agent.

ORAL ANTICOAGULANTS

WARFARIN — Warfarin is effective for treatment and secondary prevention of VTE and can be used in patients with renal impairment, but it can take up to 7 days to achieve a full therapeutic effect. Other drawbacks include dietary restrictions, drug interactions, variability in dosage requirements, and the need for close monitoring to keep the INR in the therapeutic range (2-3).

DIRECT ORAL ANTICOAGULANTS (DOACs) — Four DOACs are now available in the US (see Table 4 for FDA-approved indications). They are effective and safe for prevention and treatment of VTE and do not require INR monitoring, but data in older patients, those with renal impairment, and those with extremely low weight are limited.[10] Apixaban

Usual Adult Prophylaxis Dosage[3]	Cost[4]
5000 units SC q8-12h	$651.00
2500-5000 IU SC once/day[6]	4491.30
30 mg SC bid or 40 mg SC once/day[6]	720.00
	1025.30
2.5 mg SC once/day[6,9,10]	2255.40
	3926.10

6. Dosage adjustments may be needed for renal impairment.
7. For extended VTE treatment in patients with cancer, the dosage is 200 IU/kg SC once/day for 30 days, followed by 150 IU/kg SC once/day for 5 months (max 18,000 IU/day).
8. Dose is 5 mg if patient weighs <50 kg, 7.5 mg if 50-100 kg, 10 mg if >100 kg.
9. Contraindicated in patients with CrCl <30 mL/min.
10. Dosage for adults weighing >50 kg. Contraindicated in patients weighing <50 kg.

and rivaroxaban appear to be safe and effective in obese patients.[11] DOACs have shorter half-lives than warfarin, increasing the risk of thrombosis with missed doses. Large clinical trials comparing DOACs with each other are lacking.

Dabigatran – In patients with acute VTE treated initially for 5-10 days with UFH or LMWH, the direct thrombin inhibitor dabigatran etexilate was as effective and safe as warfarin in preventing recurrent VTE.[12] For extended treatment of VTE, dabigatran was noninferior to warfarin and had a lower risk of major bleeding.[13] There have been multiple reports of severe, sometimes fatal bleeding with dabigatran; a postmarketing study conducted by the FDA in >134,000 patients ≥65 years old, found that the risks of intracranial bleeding and death were lower with dabigatran than with warfarin, but the risk of major GI bleeding was higher with dabigatran.[14]

Table 2. Some Oral Anticoagulants for VTE[1]	
Drug	**Usual Adult Treatment Dosage**
Vitamin K Antagonist	
Warfarin[4] – generic Jantoven (USL)	2-10 mg once/day[5,6]
Direct Thrombin Inhibitor	
Dabigatran etexilate[7] – Pradaxa (Boehringer Ingelheim)	150 mg bid[8-11]
Factor Xa Inhibitors	
Apixaban – Eliquis (BMS)	10 mg bid x 7 days, then 5 mg bid[12-14]
Edoxaban – Savaysa (Daiichi-Sankyo)	60 mg once/day[8,11,15]
Rivaroxaban – Xarelto (Janssen)	15 mg bid x 3 weeks, then 20 mg once/day[8,12,16-19]

1. See Table 4 on pages 204-205 for FDA-approved VTE indications.
2. Prophylaxis is recommended for a minimum of 10-14 days and for up to 35 days after major orthopedic surgery (Y Falck-Ytter et al. Chest 2012; 141:e278S).
3. Approximate WAC for 30 days' treatment at the lowest usual adult dosage for treatment. WAC = wholesaler acquisition cost or manufacturer's published price to wholesalers; WAC represents a published catalogue or list price and may not represent an actual transactional price. Source: AnalySource® Monthly. July 5, 2022. Reprinted with permission by First Databank, Inc. All rights reserved. ©2022. www.fdbhealth.com/policies/drug-pricing-policy.
4. Coumadin is no longer being manufactured.
5. Monitor daily and adjust dose until INR is in therapeutic range (INR 2-3).
6. Requires overlap with low-molecular-weight heparin (LMWH), fondaparinux, or unfractionated heparin (UFH) for ≥5 days and until INR is ≥2 for at least 24 hours.
7. Dabigatran etexilate capsules should be stored in the original container and any remaining capsules should be discarded 4 months after opening.
8. Dosage adjustments may be needed for renal impairment.
9. Avoid coadministration with P-glycoprotein (P-gp) inhibitors in patients with CrCl <50 mL/min.

Rivaroxaban – In clinical trials, the direct factor Xa inhibitor rivaroxaban was noninferior to enoxaparin followed by a vitamin K antagonist for treatment of acute VTE, with no increase in the composite of major or clinically relevant nonmajor bleeding.[15,16] Rivaroxaban was more effective than enoxaparin in preventing VTE and death after elective hip or knee arthroplasty, but it had a higher risk of major and clinically relevant nonmajor bleeding.[17]

Apixaban – In a 6-month, randomized, double-blind trial in 5395 patients with acute VTE, the direct factor Xa inhibitor apixaban was noninferior to enoxaparin plus warfarin in preventing recurrent VTE or VTE-related

Usual Adult Prophylaxis Dosage[2]	Cost[3]
2-10 mg once/day[5,6]	$6.60
	11.10
110 mg once, then 220 mg once/day[8-10]	496.00
2.5 mg bid[12,13]	529.00
Not an FDA-approved indication	389.10
10 mg once/day[8,12,16]	516.60

10. Should not be used in patients with CrCl <30 mL/min.
11. FDA-approved for treatment of VTE following 5-10 days of initial treatment with a parenteral anticoagulant.
12. Standard doses of apixaban or rivaroxaban can be used for patients with BMI >40 kg/m[2] or weight >120 kg (KA Martin et al. J Thromb Haemost 2021; 19:1874).
13. When coadministered with a dual P-gp/strong CYP3A4 inhibitor, reduce dose by 50%; patients taking 2.5 mg bid should not take dual P-gp/strong CYP3A4 inhibitors.
14. For extended treatment after at least 3-6 months of treatment for DVT or PE, the dosage for reduction in risk of recurrence of VTE is 2.5 mg bid.
15. Dosage is 30 mg once/day in patients taking a P-gp inhibitor concurrently or who weigh ≤60 kg.
16. Should not be used in patients with CrCl <15 mL/min.
17. Avoid coadministration with dual P-gp/strong CYP3A4 inhibitors or inducers. In patients with CrCl 15-<80 mL/min, avoid coadministration with dual P-gp/moderate CYP3A4 inhibitors.
18. For extended treatment after at least 3-6 months of treatment for DVT or PE, the dosage for reduction in risk of recurrence of VTE is 10 mg once/day.
19. The 15- and 20-mg doses should be taken with food to increase bioavailability.

death, and major bleeding occurred less frequently with apixaban.[18] In two randomized controlled trials, apixaban was more effective than enoxaparin in preventing VTE or death after knee or hip replacement, with no increase in major or other clinically relevant bleeding.[19,20]

Edoxaban – In a randomized, double-blind trial in 8240 patients with acute VTE treated initially with UFH or enoxaparin, the once-daily direct factor Xa inhibitor edoxaban was noninferior to warfarin in preventing recurrent VTE or VTE-related death, and patients taking edoxaban had a significantly lower rate of major or clinically relevant nonmajor bleeding.[21]

Table 3. Duration of Anticoagulation for VTE[1]		
VTE	Recurrence Rate[2]	Duration of Anticoagulation[3]
Provoked by major transient risk factor[4]	3%[5]	3 months
Provoked by minor transient risk factor[6]	15%	3 months
Unprovoked	30%	>3 months[7]
Cancer-associated	15%[8]	>3 months

1. S Stevens et al. Chest 2021; 160:e545.
2. At 5 years.
3. >3 months (extended treatment) means there is no scheduled stop date.
4. Major transient risk factors include surgery with general anesthesia for >30 minutes, confinement to a hospital bed for ≥3 days with an acute illness, cesarean section, major trauma.
5. Recurrence of VTE provoked by surgery, a major transient risk factor.
6. Minor transient risk factors include surgery with general anesthesia for <30 minutes, hospital admission for <3 days with an acute illness, estrogen therapy, pregnancy or puerperium, confined to a non-hospital bed for ≥3 days with an acute illness, leg injury associated with reduced mobility for ≥3 days, prolonged car or air travel.
7. Risk of bleeding and risk of recurrent VTE should be considered when offering extended (>3 months) anticoagulant therapy to patients with unprovoked VTE.
8. Annualized risk of recurrence. Recurrence at 5 years not estimated because of cancer-associated mortality.

CHOICE OF ANTICOAGULANTS — Apixaban or rivaroxaban is now often preferred over parenteral anticoagulants for initial treatment of VTE. A DOAC (apixaban, dabigatran, edoxaban, or rivaroxaban) is recommended over warfarin for long-term treatment of VTE. Studies have shown that DOACs are similar to warfarin in efficacy with a lower risk of intracranial bleeding.[22] No large trials directly comparing the DOACs with each other have been published. Indirect evidence suggests that apixaban may have the lowest rate of major bleeding and may be more effective than rivaroxaban for secondary prevention of VTE.[23,24]

The 2021 CHEST guidelines recommend a factor Xa inhibitor (apixaban, edoxaban, or rivaroxaban) for initial and long-term treatment of VTE in **patients with active cancer**, who generally have a higher risk of recurrence and major bleeding.[1] In a meta-analysis of 4 randomized controlled trials that included 2894 patients with cancer, VTE recurred in

5.2% of patients treated with a factor Xa inhibitor and in 8.2% of those treated with the LMWH dalteparin.[25] The risk of major bleeding was not significantly higher with factor Xa inhibitors than with LMWH (4.3% vs 3.3%).[26,27] The risk of GI bleeding appears to be higher with edoxaban and rivaroxaban than with LMWH in patients with a luminal GI malignancy; apixaban or LMWH is preferred in such patients.[1,26,28]

For patients with **severe renal impairment** (CrCl <30 mL/min), UFH, warfarin, or apixaban is recommended for treatment of VTE.[29] In patients with nonvalvular atrial fibrillation and **normal renal function** (CrCl >95 mL/min), edoxaban was associated with an increased risk of ischemic stroke compared to warfarin; the labeling warns against its use in such patients.

Warfarin is recommended for patients with **antiphospholipid syndrome**; these patients have had a higher risk of thrombosis and stroke when treated with apixaban or rivaroxaban.[30,31]

Dabigatran, which has been associated with an increased risk of acute coronary events, is not recommended for treatment of VTE in patients with **coronary artery disease**.[27]

INR monitoring of warfarin is unreliable in patients who have **chronic liver disease** and an elevated baseline INR level.[32] LMWH is preferred in such patients. DOACs should be avoided in patients with **severe hepatic impairment**.

DURATION OF ANTICOAGULATION — The recommended duration of anticoagulant treatment for acute VTE in patients without a contraindication is 3 months. After 3 months, use of extended treatment (>3 months and sometimes indefinitely) should be considered based on the risk of VTE recurrence and bleeding. Guidelines recommend offering extended treatment to patients with unprovoked VTE or VTE provoked by a persistent risk factor such as cancer (see Table 3).[1,2]

Table 4. FDA-Approved Indications for Use of Anticoagulants in Adults with VTE

Heparin

Unfractionated Heparin
► Prophylaxis and treatment of DVT and PE

Low-Molecular-Weight Heparins (LMWHs)

Enoxaparin (*Lovenox*, and generics)
► Prophylaxis of DVT following abdominal surgery or hip or knee replacement surgery
► Prophylaxis of DVT in medical patients with severely restricted mobility during acute illness
► Treatment of acute DVT (without PE in outpatients and with or without PE in inpatients)

Dalteparin (*Fragmin*)
► Prophylaxis of DVT following abdominal surgery or hip replacement surgery
► Prophylaxis of DVT in medical patients with severely restricted mobility during acute illness
► Reduction in the risk of recurrent symptomatic VTE in cancer patients (extended treatment for 6 months)

Parenteral Factor Xa Inhibitor

Fondaparinux (*Arixtra*, and generics)
► Prophylaxis of DVT following hip fracture surgery, hip or knee replacement surgery, or abdominal surgery
► Treatment of acute DVT or PE in combination with warfarin

Vitamin K Antagonist

Warfarin
► Prophylaxis and treatment of DVT and PE

Direct Oral Anticoagulants (DOACs)

Apixaban (*Eliquis*)
► Prophylaxis of DVT following hip or knee replacement surgery
► Treatment of DVT and PE
► Reduction in the risk of recurrent DVT and PE following initial treatment lasting at least 6 months

Dabigatran etexilate (*Pradaxa*)
► Prophylaxis of DVT and PE following hip replacement surgery
► Treatment of DVT and PE following 5-10 days of initial therapy with a parenteral anticoagulant
► Reduction in the risk of recurrent DVT and PE following initial therapy

Continued on next page

Table 4. FDA-Approved Indications for Use of Anticoagulants in Adults with VTE (continued)
Direct Oral Anticoagulants (DOACs) (continued)
Edoxaban *(Savaysa)* ► Treatment of DVT and PE following 5-10 days of initial therapy with a parenteral anticoagulant
Rivaroxaban *(Xarelto)* ► Prophylaxis of DVT following hip or knee replacement surgery ► Treatment of DVT and PE ► Reduction in the risk of recurrent DVT and/or PE following initial treatment lasting at least 6 months ► Prophylaxis of VTE in acutely ill medical patients at risk for thromboembolic complications due to moderate or severe restricted mobility and other risk factors for VTE and who are not at high risk of bleeding

EXTENDED TREATMENT — There is a risk of VTE recurrence when anticoagulants are stopped. To reduce the risk, extended treatment with a low dose of a DOAC or aspirin can be considered.[1,33]

Aspirin – Two randomized, double-blind trials examined the efficacy and safety of extended treatment with aspirin after a first unprovoked VTE. In a double-blind trial, 402 patients who had completed 6 to 18 months of oral anticoagulant treatment received extended treatment for 2 years with aspirin 100 mg or placebo; the annual VTE recurrence rate was significantly lower with aspirin than with placebo (6.6% vs 11.2%). There was only one major bleeding episode in each group.[34] A double-blind, placebo-controlled trial in 822 patients who had completed initial anticoagulant treatment for a first unprovoked VTE compared aspirin 100 mg to placebo for 4 years; the rate of a composite of VTE, MI, stroke, major bleeding, or death was 33% lower in patients who received aspirin, and there were no significant differences between the two groups in bleeding rates.[35] The 2021 CHEST guidelines concluded that aspirin is not a reasonable alternative to an anticoagulant for extended treatment of VTE, but aspirin can reduce the recurrence rate in patients who are no longer taking an anticoagulant.[1]

Table 5. Non-Bleeding Adverse Effects and Drug Interactions of Anticoagulants for VTE

Drug	Some Adverse Effects
Parenteral Anticoagulants	
Unfractionated heparin (UFH)	Heparin-induced thrombocytopenia, skin necrosis, urticaria, increased liver transaminases, osteoporosis with long-term use
Enoxaparin	Thrombocytopenia, anemia, diarrhea, edema, confusion, nausea, increased serum aminotransferases, injection-site reactions (pain, bleeding, hematoma), fever
Dalteparin	Thrombocytopenia, increased serum transaminases, injection-site reactions (pain, bleeding, hematoma), skin necrosis, fever, pruritus, rash
Fondaparinux	Anemia, hypotension, insomnia, dizziness, confusion, hypokalemia, purpura, thrombocytopenia, increased serum transaminases, epistaxis
Oral Anticoagulants	
Warfarin	Vasculitis, chills, alopecia, pruritus, urticaria, abdominal pain, bloating, nausea, vomiting, diarrhea, skin necrosis
Apixaban	Epistaxis, nausea, increased serum transaminases, anemia
Dabigatran	Dyspepsia and gastritis-like symptoms
Edoxaban	Rash, abnormal liver function tests, anemia
Rivaroxaban	Abdominal pain, fatigue, back pain, muscle spasms, dizziness, anxiety, depression, insomnia, pruritus, wound secretion, UTI, increased serum transaminases

ACE = angiotensin-converting enzyme; ARB = angiotensin receptor blocker; NSAIDs = nonsteroidal anti-inflammatory drugs; P-gp = P-glycoprotein; UTI = urinary tract infection

1. Lists are not all-inclusive. Acetaminophen, amiodarone, cefazolin, cefotetan, ceftriaxone, clarithromycin, fluconazole, fluoroquinolones, fluorouracil, fluoxetine, fluvastatin, fluvoxamine, metronidazole, phenytoin (initial use), rosuvastatin, trimethoprim-sulfamethoxazole, and voriconazole can increase the anticoagulant effect of warfarin. Barbiturates, carbamazepine, cholestyramine, colestipol, dicloxacillin, nafcillin, phenytoin, rifampin, St. John's wort, and sucralfate can decrease the anticoagulant effect of warfarin.

Some Drug Interactions

Aspirin can increase the risk of bleeding/bruising; antiplatelet drugs can increase the risk of bleeding; NSAIDs can increase the anticoagulant effect; estrogens and progestins can reduce the anticoagulant effect; UFH, enoxaparin, and dalteparin may increase the hyperkalemic effects of ARBs, ACE inhibitors, potassium-sparing diuretics, aliskiren, and canagliflozin

Numerous drug and food interactions[1]

Substrate of CYP3A4 and P-gp; interacts with inhibitors and inducers of CYP3A4 and P-gp[2]; NSAIDs and other antiplatelet drugs can increase the risk of bleeding and NSAIDs may have a prothrombotic effect

Substrate of P-gp; interacts with inhibitors and inducers of P-gp[2]; NSAIDs and other antiplatelet drugs can increase the risk of bleeding and NSAIDs may have a prothrombotic effect

Substrate of P-gp; interacts with inhibitors of P-gp[2]; should not be used with the P-gp inducer rifampin; NSAIDs and other antiplatelet drugs can increase the risk of bleeding and NSAIDs may have a prothrombotic effect

Substrate of CYP3A4 and P-gp; interacts with inhibitors and inducers of CYP3A4 and P-gp[2]; NSAIDs and other antiplatelet drugs can increase the risk of bleeding and NSAIDs may have a prothrombotic effect

2. Inhibitors and inducers of CYP enzymes, P-glycoprotein, and other transporters. Med Lett Drugs Ther 2020; 62:e152.

Apixaban – In a randomized, double-blind, 12-month trial in 2482 patients with VTE who had completed 6-12 months of anticoagulation therapy, symptomatic VTE recurred in 1.7% of those taking apixaban 2.5 mg (half the usual treatment dose), 1.7% of those taking apixaban 5 mg, and 8.8% of those taking placebo. Rates of major bleeding were 0.2% with apixaban 2.5 mg, 0.1% with apixaban 5 mg, and 0.5% with placebo.[36]

Rivaroxaban – In a randomized, double-blind, 12-month trial in 3365 patients with VTE who had completed 6-12 months of anticoagulation therapy, a symptomatic VTE recurred in 1.2% of patients taking rivaroxaban 10 mg (half the usual treatment dose), 1.5% of those taking rivaroxaban 20 mg, and 4.4% of those taking aspirin 100 mg. Rates of major bleeding were 0.4% with rivaroxaban 10 mg, 0.5% with rivaroxaban 20 mg, and 0.3% with aspirin.[37]

ADVERSE EFFECTS — The major adverse effect of all anticoagulants is bleeding, especially intracranial bleeding, which occurs about half as often with DOACs as it does with warfarin.[38] Nonbleeding adverse effects are summarized in Table 5.

DRUG INTERACTIONS — Many drugs can increase the risk of bleeding when coadministered with anticoagulants. Some drug interactions are listed in Table 5.

PRIMARY PREVENTION OF VTE — LMWH has generally been recommended for orthopedic and nonorthopedic surgery patients for whom postoperative prophylaxis is indicated.[4-6] Recent guidelines recommend a DOAC or aspirin for prevention of VTE in patients undergoing total hip or knee replacement surgery.[6] Rivaroxaban and apixaban are as effective as LMWH for prevention of VTE after knee or hip replacement surgery,[39-41] but the risk of bleeding may be higher with rivaroxaban.[42] In a double-blind trial, 3424 patients undergoing total hip or knee arthroplasty received once-daily rivaroxaban 10 mg for 5 days postoperatively and were then randomized to receive either rivaroxaban or aspirin 81 mg daily for an additional 9 days (total knee arthroplasty) or 30 days (total hip arthroplasty). Symptomatic VTE occurred in 0.64% of patients taking aspirin and in 0.70% of those taking rivaroxaban. Rates of major bleeding were 0.47% with aspirin and 0.29% with rivaroxaban. None of these differences were statistically significant.[43]

For prevention of VTE in hospitalized medical patients who are at increased risk of thrombosis, LMWH, low-dose UFH, or fondaparinux has been recommended.[7] Rivaroxaban is FDA-approved for this indication, but in a meta-analysis of randomized controlled trials, use of a DOAC did not reduce the risk of VTE compared to LMWH and the risk of major bleeding was higher.[44]

REVERSAL OF ANTICOAGULATION — In patients with serious bleeding caused by UFH, IV infusion of **protamine** can be used to reverse the anticoagulant effect. IV protamine is less effective for reversal of the anticoagulant effect of LMWH; andexanet alfa (see below) may be preferred.[45,46] For patients with bleeding caused by warfarin, treatment with **vitamin K** can normalize the INR in 12-24 hours; for major bleeding or emergent surgery, 4-factor prothrombin complex concentrate is recommended as well.[47] *Kcentra*, a human derived 4-factor **prothrombin complex concentrate** is FDA-approved for urgent reversal of warfarin anticoagulation in adults with acute major bleeding.[48]

Idarucizumab *(Praxbind)*, a humanized monoclonal antibody fragment, is FDA-approved for urgent reversal of the anticoagulant effect of the direct thrombin inhibitor dabigatran.[49] Idarucizumab rapidly decreases circulating levels of unbound dabigatran, neutralizing its anticoagulant effect within minutes. In a clinical trial, the median time to cessation of bleeding was ~2.5 hours.[50] Reversal with idarucizumab persists for 12-24 hours.

Andexanet alfa *(Andexxa)*, a recombinant human factor Xa decoy protein that binds factor Xa inhibitors, is FDA-approved for urgent reversal of the anticoagulant effect of apixaban and rivaroxaban. In a clinical trial, a bolus and subsequent 2-hour infusion of the drug markedly reduced anti-factor Xa activity.[51-53] Andexanet alfa has been used off-label for reversal of the anticoagulant effect of other factor Xa inhibitors as well.[54] It also reverses the anticoagulant effect of LMWH.[45-46] Reversal with andexanet alfa lasts only about 2 hours.

The results of some studies indicate that the anticoagulant effects of DOACs can be reversed by prothrombin complex concentrates.[50]

PREGNANCY AND LACTATION — **UFH** has been used safely in pregnant women for many years. The large heparin molecule does not cross the placenta and, unlike warfarin, the drug is not teratogenic or toxic to the fetus. **LMWH** appears to be at least as safe and effective as UFH, and it is less likely to cause osteoporosis or heparin-induced thrombocytopenia[55]; LMWH is recommended for use during pregnancy. Data on use of **fondaparinux** during pregnancy are limited; its use is generally reserved for patients unable to use LMWH. **DOACs** should not be used in pregnant women; some have caused fetal toxicity in animal studies. DOACs may be excreted in human breast milk and should be avoided in women who are breastfeeding. **Warfarin** should not be used during pregnancy, but it appears to be safe for use in women who are breastfeeding.

COVID-19 — COVID-19 has been associated with inflammation and a prothrombotic state. In one meta-analysis, the prevalence of VTE in hospitalized patients with COVID-19 was 14%.[56] Multiple organizations have published guidelines on the use of antithrombotic therapy in COVID-19.[57-59]

1. TL Ortel et al. American Society of Hematology 2020 guidelines for management of venous thromboembolism: treatment of deep vein thrombosis and pulmonary embolism. Blood Adv 2020; 4:4693.
2. SM Stevens et al. Antithrombotic therapy for VTE disease: second update of the CHEST guideline and expert panel report. Chest 2021; 160:e545.
3. CD Jackson et al. Antithrombotic therapy for venous thromboembolism. JAMA 2022; 327:2141.
4. Y Falck-Ytter et al. Prevention of VTE in orthopedic surgery patients: antithrombotic therapy and prevention of thrombosis, 9th ed: American College of Chest Physicians evidence-based clinical practice guidelines. Chest 2012; 141(2 Suppl):e278S.

5. MK Gould et al. Prevention of VTE in nonorthopedic surgical patients: antithrombotic therapy and prevention of thrombosis, 9th ed: American College of Chest Physicians evidence-based clinical practice guidelines. Chest 2012; 141(2 Suppl):e227S.

6. DR Anderson et al. American Society of Hematology 2019 guidelines for management of venous thromboembolism: prevention of venous thromboembolism in surgical hospitalized patients. Blood Adv 2019; 3:3898.

7. HJ Schünemann et al. American Society of Hematology 2018 guidelines for management of venous thromboembolism: prophylaxis for hospitalized and non-hospitalized medical patients. Blood Adv 2018; 2:3198.

8. C Wall et al. Catheter-related thrombosis: a practical approach. J Intensive Care Soc 2016; 17:160.

9. SA Smith et al. How it all starts: initiation of the clotting cascade. Crit Rev Biochem Mol Biol 2015; 50:326.

10. New oral anticoagulants for acute venous thromboembolism. Med Lett Drugs Ther 2014; 56:3.

11. KA Martin et al. Use of direct oral anticoagulants in patients with obesity for treatment and prevention of venous thromboembolism: updated communication from the ISTH SSC subcommittee on control of anticoagulation. J Thromb Haemost 2021; 19:1874.

12. S Schulman et al. Dabigatran versus warfarin in the treatment of acute venous thromboembolism. N Engl J Med 2009; 361:2342.

13. S Schulman et al. Extended use of dabigatran, warfarin, or placebo in venous thromboembolism. N Engl J Med 2013; 368:709.

14. FDA Drug Safety Communication: FDA study of medicare patients finds risks lower for stroke and death but higher for gastrointestinal bleeding with Pradaxa (dabigatran) compared to warfarin. May 13, 2014. Available at: https://bit.ly/3ydIXAG. Accessed July 7, 2022.

15. EINSTEIN Investigators et al. Oral rivaroxaban for symptomatic venous thromboembolism. N Engl J Med 2010; 363:2499.

16. EINSTEIN-PE Investigators et al. Oral rivaroxaban for the treatment of symptomatic pulmonary embolism. N Engl J Med 2012; 366:1287.

17. Rivaroxaban (Xarelto) – a new oral anticoagulant. Med Lett Drugs Ther 2011; 53:65.

18. G Agnelli et al. Oral apixaban for the treatment of acute venous thromboembolism. N Engl J Med 2013; 369:799.

19. MR Lassen et al. Apixaban versus enoxaparin for thromboprophylaxis after knee replacement (ADVANCE-2): a randomised double-blind trial. Lancet 2010; 375:807.

20. MR Lassen et al. Apixaban versus enoxaparin for thromboprophylaxis after hip replacement. N Engl J Med 2010; 363:2487.

21. Hokusai-VTE Investigators et al. Edoxaban versus warfarin for the treatment of symptomatic venous thromboembolism. N Engl J Med 2013; 369:1406.

22. N van Es et al. Direct oral anticoagulants compared with vitamin K antagonists for acute venous thromboembolism: evidence from phase 3 trials. Blood 2014; 124:1968.

23. N Kang and DM Sobieraj. Indirect treatment comparison of new oral anticoagulants for the treatment of acute venous thromboembolism. Thromb Res 2014; 133:1145.

24. GK Dawwas et al. Risk for recurrent venous thromboembolism and bleeding with apixaban compared with rivaroxaban: an analysis of real-world data. Ann Intern Med 2022; 175:20.

25. M Giustozzi et al. Direct oral anticoagulants for the treatment of acute venous thromboembolism associated with cancer: a systematic review and meta-analysis. Thromb Haemost 2020; 120:1128.

26. G Agnelli et al. Apixaban for the treatment of venous thromboembolism associated with cancer. N Engl J Med 2020; 382:1599.

27. K Uchino and AV Hernandez. Dabigatran association with higher risk of acute coronary events: meta-analysis of noninferiority randomized controlled trials. Arch Intern Med 2012; 172:397.

28. AYY Lee. Anticoagulant therapy for venous thromboembolism in cancer. N Engl J Med 2020; 382:1650.

29. CYS Cheung et al. Direct oral anticoagulant use in chronic kidney disease and dialysis patients with venous thromboembolism: a systematic review of thrombosis and bleeding outcomes. Ann Pharmacother 2021: 55:711.

30. J Ordi-Ros et al. Rivaroxaban versus vitamin K antagonist in antiphospholipid syndrome: a randomized noninferiority trial. Ann Intern Med 2019; 171:685.

31. SC Woller et al. Apixaban compared with warfarin to prevent thrombosis in thrombotic antiphospholipid syndrome: a randomized trial. Blood Adv 2022; 6:1661.

32. A Dhar et al. Anticoagulation in chronic liver disease. J Hepatol 2017; 66:1313.

33. L Vasanthamohan et al. Reduced-dose direct oral anticoagulants in the extended treatment of venous thromboembolism: a systematic review and meta-analysis. J Thromb Haemost 2018; 16:1288.

34. C Becattini et al. Aspirin for preventing the recurrence of venous thromboembolism. N Engl J Med 2012; 366:1959.

35. TA Brighton et al. Low-dose aspirin for preventing recurrent venous thromboembolism. N Engl J Med 2012; 367:1979.

36. G Agnelli et al. Apixaban for extended treatment of venous thromboembolism. N Engl J Med 2013; 368:699.

37. JI Weitz et al. Rivaroxaban or aspirin for extended treatment of venous thromboembolism. N Engl J Med 2017; 376:1211.

38. Which oral anticoagulant for atrial fibrillation? Med Lett Drugs Ther 2016; 58:45.

39. MR Lassen et al. Rivaroxaban versus enoxaparin for thromboprophylaxis after total knee arthroplasty. N Engl J Med 2008; 358:2776.

40. MR Lassen et al. Apixaban versus enoxaparin for thromboprophylaxis after hip replacement. N Engl J Med 2010; 363:2487.

41. T Haykal et al. Thromboprophylaxis for orthopedic surgery; an updated meta-analysis. Thromb Res 2021; 199:43.

42. BT Venker et al. Safety and efficacy of new anticoagulants for the prevention of venous thromboembolism after hip and knee arthroplasty: a meta-analysis. J Arthroplasty 2017; 32:645.

43. DR Anderson et al. Aspirin or rivaroxaban for VTE prophylaxis after hip or knee arthroplasty. N Engl J Med 2018; 378:699.

44. I Neumann et al. DOACs vs LMWHs in hospitalized medical patients: a systematic review and meta-analysis that informed 2018 ASH guidelines. Blood Adv 2020; 4:1512.

45. S Kaatz et al. Reversing factor Xa inhibitors – clinical utility of andexanet alfa. J Blood Med 2017; 8:141.

46. E Carpenter et al. Andexanet alfa for reversal of factor Xa inhibitor-associated anticoagulation. Ther Adv Drug Saf 2019 Nov 26 (epub).
47. S Christos and R Naples. Anticoagulation reversal and treatment strategies in major bleeding: update 2016. West J Emerg Med 2016; 17:264.
48. Kcentra: a 4-factor prothrombin complex concentrate for reversal of warfarin anticoagulation. Med Lett Drugs Ther 2013; 55:53.
49. Idarucizumab (Praxbind) – an antidote for dabigatran. Med Lett Drugs Ther 2015; 57:157.
50. CV Pollack Jr. et al. Idarucizumab for dabigatran reversal – full cohort analysis. N Engl J Med 2017; 377:431.
51. Andexxa – an antidote for apixaban and rivaroxaban. Med Lett Drugs Ther 2018; 60:99.
52. SJ Connolly et al. Full study report of andexanet alfa for bleeding associated with factor Xa inhibitors. N Engl J Med 2019; 380:1326.
53. SJ Connolly et al. Andexanet alfa for acute major bleeding associated with factor Xa inhibitors. N Engl J Med 2016; 375:1131.
54. GF Tomaselli et al. 2020 ACC expert consensus decision pathway on management of bleeding in patients on oral anticoagulants: a report of the American College of Cardiology Solution Set Oversight Committee. J Am Coll Cardiol 2020; 76:594.
55. SM Bates et al. American Society of Hematology 2018 guidelines for management of venous thromboembolism in the context of pregnancy. Blood Adv 2018; 2:3317.
56. S Nopp et al. Risk of venous thromboembolism in patients with COVID-19: a systematic review and meta-analysis. Res Pract Thromb Haemost 2020; 4:1178.
57. COVID-19 Treatment Guidelines Panel. Coronavirus disease 2019 (COVID-19) treatment guidelines. National Institutes of Health. Available at: https://bit.ly/3w2faYJ. Accessed July 7, 2022.
58. LK Moores et al. Thromboprophylaxis in patients with COVID-19: a brief update to the CHEST guideline and expert panel report. Chest 2022 Feb 12 (epub).
59. A Cuker et al. American Society of Hematology living guidelines on the use of anticoagulation for thromboprophylaxis in patients with COVID-19: January 2022 update on the use of therapeutic-intensity anticoagulation in acutely ill patients. Blood Adv 2022 May 3 (epub).

DRUGS AND DEVICES FOR
Weight Management

Original publication date – May 2022

Adults with a body mass index (BMI) between 25 and 29.9 kg/m^2 are considered overweight. Those with a BMI ≥30 are considered obese. The initial recommendation for any weight loss effort is to achieve a 5-10% reduction in weight, which has been associated with a reduction in the risk of developing type 2 diabetes, hypertension, and dyslipidemia. Diet, exercise, and behavior modification are the preferred methods for losing weight, but long-term weight maintenance can be difficult. Several drugs and devices are FDA-approved for weight reduction and maintenance of weight loss.

DRUGS

Pharmacologic therapy should be reserved for adults with a BMI ≥30 kg/m^2 or a BMI ≥27 and at least one weight-related comorbidity, such as hypertension, dyslipidemia, cardiovascular disease, obstructive sleep apnea, or type 2 diabetes, who have not achieved ≥5% weight loss with lifestyle modification. All weight-loss drugs have been associated with weight regain when the drug is stopped.

SYMPATHOMIMETIC AMINES — The oldest weight-loss drugs are sympathomimetic amines such as phentermine (*Adipex-P*, and others) and diethylpropion, which are FDA-approved only for short-term use (up to 12 weeks). Most studies have reported additional weight loss of only

Drugs and Devices for Weight Management

Summary: Drugs and Devices for Weight Management

▶ Diet, exercise, and behavior modification are the preferred methods for losing weight.

▶ Pharmacologic therapy should be reserved for adults with a BMI $\geq$30 kg/m^2 or a BMI $\geq$27 and at least one weight-related comorbidity who have not achieved $\geq$5% weight loss with lifestyle modification.

▶ The most effective drugs for weight loss are oral phentermine/topiramate (*Qsymia*) and subcutaneously injected semaglutide (*Wegovy*).

▶ For patients who can tolerate once-weekly injections, semaglutide (*Wegovy*) is preferred.

▶ Intragastric balloon devices (*Orbera* and *Obalon*) have limited long-term efficacy.

▶ Weight-loss drugs and devices are contraindicated for use during pregnancy.

a fraction of a pound per week in patients taking these drugs compared to placebo-treated patients. In an electronic health record cohort study, patients with a BMI $\geq$27 kg/m^2 who consistently used phentermine for >12 months achieved significantly more weight loss than those who took the drug for <3 months (-7.4% vs -0.2%). There was no difference in cardiovascular-related adverse events between the cohorts, but patients with pre-existing cardiovascular disease were excluded from the analysis.[1]

Qsymia, a fixed-dose combination of phentermine and an extended-release formulation of the antiseizure drug topiramate approved for use in adults, has produced a dose-dependent mean weight loss of 6-13 kg (6 kg with 3.75/23 mg and 13 kg with 15/92 mg) over 56 weeks, and 70% of patients treated with the higher dose achieved $\geq$5% weight loss, with little regression to baseline over 2 years of continuous use.[2-4] In a meta-analysis that included 143 trials of weight-loss drugs in a total of 49,810 participants, phentermine/topiramate was the most effective oral drug in achieving weight loss.[5]

In a randomized, double-blind trial in 227 obese adolescents (12 to 16 years old), the estimated mean change from baseline in BMI at 56 weeks was significantly greater with phentermine/topiramate than with placebo (-4.8% with 7.5/46 mg and -7.1% with 15/92 mg vs -3.3%

with placebo).[6] To date, the combination has not been approved by the FDA for use in adolescents.

If ≥5% weight loss is not achieved after 12 weeks on the maximum dose of *Qsymia*, the drug should be stopped gradually; abrupt discontinuation of topiramate can cause seizures, even in patients with no history of seizures. Unlike phentermine alone, *Qsymia* is FDA-approved for use beyond 3 months. Data on cardiovascular outcomes with the combination are not available.

Adverse Effects – All sympathomimetic amines can increase heart rate and blood pressure and cause nervousness. Phentermine/topiramate can cause dry mouth, paresthesia, constipation, dysgeusia, and insomnia. Impairment of cognition, attention, concentration, and memory has also been reported. Topiramate is a carbonic anhydrase inhibitor and can cause metabolic acidosis, which increases the risk of kidney stones. *Qsymia* is a schedule IV controlled substance and is only available through a REMS program designed to prevent its use during pregnancy. Other contraindications to its use are listed in Table 4.

Drug Interactions – Use of sympathomimetic amines are contraindicated with or within 14 days of a monoamine oxidase inhibitor.

ORLISTAT — Available both over the counter *(Alli)* and by prescription *(Xenical)*, orlistat is a pancreatic and gastric lipase inhibitor that decreases GI absorption of fat. Unlike other weight-loss drugs, low-dose orlistat *(Alli)* is approved for patients with a BMI ≥25 kg/m^2. In a meta-analysis that included 143 trials of weight-loss drugs in a total of 49,810 participants, orlistat was minimally effective in achieving weight loss (-3.1%) and had a high incidence of GI adverse effects leading to drug discontinuation.[5]

Adverse Effects – Flatulence with discharge, oily spotting, and fecal urgency can occur in patients taking orlistat, mainly after consumption of high-fat foods. Severe liver injury has been reported rarely, but a causal

Table 1. Dosage and Cost of FDA-Approved Drugs for Weight Management[1]

Drug	Some Available Formulations
Sympathomimetic Amines	
Benzphetamine – generic	50 mg tabs
Diethylpropion – generic	25 mg tabs
extended-release – generic	75 mg ER tabs
Phendimetrazine – generic	35 mg tabs
extended-release – generic	105 mg ER caps
Phentermine[5] – generic	15, 30, 37.5 mg caps; 37.5 mg tabs
Adipex-P (Teva)	37.5 mg caps, tabs
Lomaira (KVK-Tech)	8 mg tabs
Sympathomimetic Amine/Antiseizure Combination	
Phentermine/topiramate ER –	3.75/23, 7.5/46, 11.25/69, 15/92 mg
Qsymia (Vivus)	ER caps
Lipase Inhibitor	
Orlistat – *Xenical* (Cheplapharm)	120 mg caps
Alli[8] (GSK)	60 mg caps
Opioid Antagonist/Antidepressant Combination	
Naltrexone/bupropion – *Contrave* (Currax)	8/90 mg ER tabs
Glucagon-Like Peptide-1 (GLP-1) Receptor Agonists	
Liraglutide – *Saxenda* (Novo Nordisk)	18 mg/3 mL prefilled pen[13]
Semaglutide – *Wegovy* (Novo Nordisk)[17]	0.25, 0.5, 1 mg/0.5 mL; 1.7, 2.4 mg/0.75 mL single-dose pens

ER = extended-release
1. Weight loss drugs, including over-the-counter medications, are contraindicated for use during pregnancy.
2. Placebo-corrected weight loss above diet and lifestyle modifications alone.
3. Approximate WAC for 30 days' treatment at the lowest usual adult dosage. WAC = wholesaler acqui- sition cost or manufacturer's published price to wholesalers; WAC represents a published catalogue or list price and may not represent an actual transactional price. Source: AnalySource® Monthly. May 5, 2022. Reprinted with permission by First Databank, Inc. All rights reserved. ©2022. www.fdbhealth. com/policies/drug-pricing-policy.
4. Only approved for short-term use (up to 12 weeks). Most studies have reported an additional weight loss of only a fraction of a pound per week compared to placebo-treated patients.
5. Phentermine was widely used with fenfluramine until the combination ("phen-fen") was found to be associated with heart valve abnormalities. Fenfluramine has been withdrawn from the market.
6. The recommended starting dosage is 3.75/23 mg in the morning for 14 days, then 7.5/46 mg for 12 weeks, and 15/72 mg thereafter. If ≥5% weight loss is not achieved after 12 weeks on the maximum dose, the drug should be stopped. *Qsymia* should be discontinued gradually.
7. DB Allison et al. Obesity 2012; 20:330; KM Gadde et al. Lancet 2011; 377:1341.
8. Available over the counter.
9. SZ Yanovski and JA Yanovski. JAMA 2014; 311:74.
10. The recommended starting dosage is 1 tablet in the morning for 7 days, then one tablet twice daily in week 2, 2 tablets in the morning and 1 in the evening in week 3, and 2 tablets in the morning and evening in week 4 and thereafter.

Usual Adult Dosage	Mean Weight Loss[2]/ % Patients with Weight Loss ≥5%	Cost[3]
25-50 mg PO once/day-tid	See Footnote 4	$37.50
25 mg PO tid	See Footnote 4	20.10
75 mg PO once/day		25.30
35 mg PO bid or tid	See Footnote 4	8.20
105 mg PO once/day		32.30
15-37.5 mg PO once/day	See Footnote 4	16.00
37.5 mg PO once/day	See Footnote 4	62.40
8 mg PO tid	See Footnote 4	43.50
7.5/46-15/92 mg PO once/day[6]	6.0-12.6 kg/45-70%[7]	
		186.00
120 mg PO tid	2.5-3.4 kg/35-73%[9]	586.10
60 mg PO tid		44.00
16/180 mg PO bid[10,11]	3.7-5.2 kg/39-66%[12]	278.00
3 mg SC once/day[14]	5.6-8.4 kg/51-63%[15,16]	1349.00
2.4 mg SC once/week[18]	7.1-16.8 kg/67-85%[15,19]	1349.00[20]

11. If ≥5% weight loss is not achieved after 12 weeks on the maximum dose, the drug should be stopped.
12. FL Greenway et al. Lancet 2010; 376:595; CM Apovian et al. Obesity 2013; 21:935; TA Wadden et al. Obesity 2011; 19:110.
13. Each pen can deliver doses of 0.6, 1.2, 1.8, 2.4, or 3 mg. Sold in packages containing 3 or 5 multi-dose pens.
14. The recommended starting dosage is 0.6 mg injected subcutaneously once/day; the dose should be increased in 0.6-mg increments each week to 2.4 mg at week 4 and to 3 mg thereafter. If the patient has not lost ≥4% of baseline body weight at week 16, liraglutide should be stopped.
15. Trials included patients with and without type 2 diabetes.
16. TA Wadden et al. Int J Obes (Lond) 2015; 39:187; X Pi-Sunyer et al. N Engl J Med 2015; 373:11; MJ Davies et al. JAMA 2015; 314:687.
17. According to the manufacturer, a shortage of the drug is expected for the first half of 2022.
18. The recommended starting dosage is 0.25 mg injected subcutaneously once weekly; the dose should be increased to 0.5 mg for weeks 5-8, 1 mg for weeks 9-12, 1.7 mg for weeks 13-16, and 2.4 mg thereafter.
19. JPH Wilding et al. N Engl J Med 2021; 384:989; TA Wadden et al. JAMA 2021; 325:1403; D Rubino et al. JAMA 2021; 325:1414; M Davies et al. Lancet 2021; 397:971.
20. Compounding pharmacies are providing semaglutide in various strengths and in combination with other agents, such as vitamin B12, at a lower cost. These formulations have not been approved by the FDA.

relationship has not been established. Orlistat increases oxalate absorption and may increase the risk of developing calcium oxalate kidney stones. Contraindications to use of orlistat are listed in Table 4.

Drug Interactions – Because orlistat reduces absorption of fat-soluble vitamins, patients taking the drug should also take a multivitamin supplement containing fat-soluble vitamins daily at bedtime.[7] Patients taking levothyroxine should take it 4 hours before or after taking orlistat. Orlistat may reduce vitamin K absorption; patients on stable doses of warfarin or other anticoagulants should be monitored for changes in coagulation parameters. Cyclosporine serum concentrations may be reduced when coadministered with orlistat; cyclosporine should be taken 3 hours after orlistat. Orlistat may reduce serum concentrations and possibly the efficacy of amiodarone. Patients taking antiretroviral drugs for HIV infection may experience a reduction in the efficacy of their antiretroviral regimen while taking orlistat; the exact mechanism is unclear.

NALTREXONE/BUPROPION — The opioid antagonist naltrexone and the dopamine/norepinephrine reuptake inhibitor bupropion are available in a fixed-dose combination *(Contrave)* that is FDA-approved for weight management. In clinical trials, the combination was associated with a 3-5% placebo-corrected weight loss, and 39-66% of patients achieved ≥5% weight loss after 56 weeks.[8,9] In a meta-analysis that included 143 trials of weight-loss drugs in a total of 49,810 participants, weight loss with naltrexone/bupropion was modest (-4.1%) and the combination had the highest incidence of adverse effects leading to drug discontinuation of all FDA-approved weight-loss drugs.[5] If ≥5% weight loss is not achieved after 12 weeks at the maintenance dosage, the drug should be stopped.

Adverse Effects – Naltrexone/bupropion can cause nausea, vomiting, headache, constipation, insomnia, dizziness, and dry mouth. The labeling includes a boxed warning about suicidal thoughts and behavior associated with use of antidepressants and serious neuropsychiatric reactions reported with use of bupropion for smoking cessation. In clinical

Table 2. Some Liraglutide Clinical Trial Results[1]		
Regimen	Mean Weight Loss (%)	% of Patients with Weight Loss ≥5%
Patients with Diabetes		
MJ Davies et al; 56 weeks (n=846)[2]		
Liraglutide 3 mg	6.0%	54.3%
Liraglutide 1.8 mg[3]	4.7%	40.4%
Placebo	2.0%	21.4%
Patients without Diabetes		
X Pi-Sunyer et al; 56 weeks (n=3731)[4]		
Liraglutide 3 mg	8.0%	63.2%
Placebo	2.6%	27.1%
Patients without Diabetes after ≥5% Initial Weight Loss[5]		
TA Wadden et al; 56 weeks (n=422)[6]		
Liraglutide 3 mg	6.2%[7]	50.5%[7]
Placebo	0.2%[7]	21.8%[7]

1. In addition to diet and exercise in adults with a BMI ≥30 or a BMI ≥27 and at least one weight-related comorbidity.
2. MJ Davies et al. JAMA 2015; 314:687.
3. FDA-approved as a titration dose, but not for maintenance.
4. X Pi-Sunyer et al. N Engl J Med 2015; 373:11.
5. Patients were first treated with a low-calorie diet and lost ≥5% of initial body weight in 4-12 weeks during the run-in phase.
6. TA Wadden et al. Int J Obes (Lond) 2013; 37:1443.
7. Weight loss observed after randomization.

trials, use of bupropion/naltrexone was not associated with suicidality. Bupropion may lower the seizure threshold. Increases in heart rate and blood pressure have been reported; the drug is not recommended for use in patients with uncontrolled hypertension.[10] Aminotransferase elevations and hepatotoxicity have been reported in patients taking naltrexone. Contraindications to use of the combination are listed in Table 4.

Drug Interactions – Use of naltrexone/bupropion is contraindicated with or within 14 days of a monoamine oxidase inhibitor. The combination can reduce the efficacy of opioid-containing drugs; naltrexone/bupropion is contraindicated for use with chronic opioid or opiate agonists or partial agonists. Naltrexone/bupropion can increase serum concentrations and

Table 3. Some Semaglutide Clinical Trial Results

Study	Regimen	Mean Weight Change (%)[1]
Patients without Type 2 Diabetes		
STEP 1[2]	Semaglutide[3]	-15.3 kg (-14.9%)*
68 weeks (n=1961)	Placebo	-2.6 kg (-2.4%)
STEP 3[4]	Semaglutide[3]	-16.8 kg (-16.0%)*
68 weeks (n=611)	Placebo	-6.2 kg (-5.7%)
STEP 4[5]	Semaglutide[6]	-7.1 kg (-7.9%)*
68 weeks (n=803)	Placebo	+6.1 kg (+6.9%)
Patients with Type 2 Diabetes		
STEP 2[7]	Semaglutide[3]	-9.7 kg (-9.6%)*
68 weeks (n=1210)	Placebo	-3.5 kg (-3.4%)

*Statistically significant difference vs placebo
1. Mean change in body weight from baseline to week 68 in STEP 1-3. Mean change in body weight from week 20-68 in STEP 4.
2. In addition to a reduced calorie diet, exercise, and counseling in adults with a BMI ≥30 or ≥27 and at least one weight-related comorbidity. JPH Wilding et al. N Engl J Med 2021; 384:989.
3. Dose was titrated over 16 weeks to reach 2.4 mg injected subcutaneously once/week. Lower maintenance doses were allowed if patients had unacceptable adverse effects with the 2.4-mg dose. STEP 2 also included a semaglutide 1.0-mg treatment arm; the 2.4-mg dose was significantly more effective at reducing body weight than the 1.0-mg dose.
4. In addition to intensive behavioral therapy plus low-calorie meal replacements (1000-1200 kcal/day) for the first 8 weeks followed by a conventional diet in adults with a BMI ≥30 or ≥27 and at least one weight-related comorbidity. TA Wadden et al. JAMA 2021; 325:1403.
5. In addition to lifestyle intervention in adults with a BMI ≥30 or ≥27 and at least one weight-related comorbidity. D Rubino et al. JAMA 2021; 325:1414.
6. Dose was titrated over 16 weeks to reach 2.4 mg once/week and then continued to week 20. Patients were then randomized to continue semaglutide treatment or switch to placebo. Lower maintenance doses were allowed if patients could not tolerate the 2.4 mg dose.
7. In addition to lifestyle intervention in adults with a BMI ≥27. M Davies et al. Lancet 2021; 397:971.

possibly the toxicity of drugs that are metabolized by CYP2D6.[11] Coadministration of the combination and digoxin may decrease serum concentrations of digoxin. Bupropion is primarily metabolized by CYP2B6; inhibitors of CYP2B6 may increase serum concentrations of bupropion and decrease hydroxybupropion exposure and inducers can reduce serum concentrations of the drug and possibly its efficacy. Bupropion may lower seizure threshold; use caution when naltrexone/bupropion is used with other drugs that lower seizure threshold. Bupropion has dopamine agonist effects; CNS toxicity has been reported when the drug was coadministered with levodopa or amantadine.

GLP-1 RECEPTOR AGONISTS — Two subcutaneously injected glucagon-like peptide-1 (GLP-1) receptor agonists, liraglutide and semaglutide, are FDA-approved for weight management in patients with and without type 2 diabetes; with both drugs, the dosage recommended for weight loss is higher than the dosage used for treatment of type 2 diabetes.

Liraglutide – The once-daily injectable GLP-1 receptor agonist liraglutide, which is FDA-approved for treatment of type 2 diabetes as *Victoza*,[12] has been available since 2014 as *Saxenda* for chronic weight management in adults with a BMI ≥30 kg/m^2 or ≥27 and at least one weight-related comorbidity.[13] *Saxenda* has recently been approved for chronic weight management in patients ≥12 years old who weigh more than 60 kg and are obese (defined by specific BMI cut-offs for age and sex that correspond to a BMI ≥30 for adults).

In placebo-controlled clinical trials in overweight and obese patients with or without diabetes, patients treated with liraglutide 3 mg once daily had a placebo-corrected weight loss of 4-5.4% (see Table 2).[14-16]

In a 3-year, randomized, double-blind trial in 1128 patients with prediabetes, use of liraglutide 3 mg/day resulted in a placebo-corrected weight loss of 4.3%.[17]

A randomized controlled trial assessed the efficacy of liraglutide 3 mg/day (with and without exercise) for weight loss maintenance by enrolling 195 obese patients without diabetes into different treatment arms after an 8-week low-calorie diet produced a mean decrease in body weight of 13.1 kg. Maintenance of weight loss through 52 weeks was better with addition of liraglutide alone (-0.7 kg) and with exercise (-3.4 kg) than with exercise alone (+2.0 kg) or placebo (+6.1 kg).[18]

Semaglutide – The once-weekly injectable GLP-1 receptor agonist semaglutide, which is FDA-approved as *Ozempic* for treatment of type 2 diabetes, has been approved in a higher dose as *Wegovy* for chronic weight management in adults with a BMI ≥30 kg/m^2 or ≥27 and at least

Table 4. Weight-Loss Drugs: Key Points	
Drug	**Comments**

Sympathomimetic Amines
  Benzphetamine
  Diethylpropion
  Phendimetrazine
  Phentermine
	► FDA-approved for short-term use (up to 12 weeks)
	► Limited data with longer use

Phentermine/topiramate ER *(Qsymia)*	► FDA-approved for use in adults; recent data in adolescents 12-16 years old ► Most effective oral weight loss drug (10.9% with 15/92 mg at 56 wks) ► Only available through a REMS program designed to prevent use during pregnancy ► Schedule IV controlled substance ► Dosage adjustments required for moderate or severe renal impairment or moderate hepatic impairment
Orlistat *(Xenical/Alli)*	► FDA-approved for short-term use in adults (up to 12 weeks) ► Available over the counter in a low dose for patients with a BMI ≥25 ► Minimally effective for weight loss (-3.1% in one meta-analysis)

Some Contraindications/Precautions

▶ Contraindications
- Pregnancy/breastfeeding
- Cardiovascular disease
- Uncontrolled hypertension
- Glaucoma
- Hyperthyroidism
- History of drug abuse/agitation
- Within 14 days of a MAOI

▶ Contraindications
- Pregnancy
- Glaucoma
- Hyperthyroidism
- Within 14 days of a MAOI

▶ Precautions
- Abrupt discontinuation can cause seizures
- Can cause fetal harm; monthly pregnancy testing required in women who can become pregnant

▶ Adverse effects requiring monitoring:
- Tachycardia
- Mood disorders/suicidal ideation
- Cognitive impairment
- Metabolic acidosis
- Increased serum creatinine
- Acute closed-angle glaucoma

▶ Contraindications
- Pregnancy
- Chronic malabsorption syndrome
- Cholestasis

▶ Precautions
- Severe hepatic injury
- Increased urinary oxalate/nephrolithiasis

Continued on next page

Table 4. Weight-Loss Drugs: Key Points (continued)	
Drug	**Comments**
Naltrexone/bupropion (*Contrave*)	► FDA-approved for use in adults ► 3-5% placebo-corrected weight loss at 56 weeks ► Dosage adjustments required for moderate or severe renal impairment or moderate hepatic impairment
GLP-1 Receptor Agonists Liraglutide (*Saxenda*) Semaglutide (*Wegovy*)	**Liraglutide** ► FDA-approved for use in adults and adolescents ≥12 years old ► Weight loss up to 8% in clinical trials ► Improved cardiovascular outcomes in patients with type 2 diabetes **Semaglutide** ► FDA-approved for use in adults ► Most effective weight-loss drug available (up to 16% in clinical trials) ► Improved cardiovascular outcomes in patients with type 2 diabetes
MAOI = monoamine oxidase inhibitor	

one weight-related comorbidity.[19] The oral formulation of semaglutide (*Rybelsus*) has not been approved for weight management.

In 3 double-blind trials (STEP 1-3) in overweight or obese adults with and without type 2 diabetes, mean weight loss from baseline to week 68 was significantly greater with semaglutide 2.4 mg once weekly than with placebo (see Table 3). In a fourth trial (STEP 4), overweight or obese adults who reached a target dose of semaglutide 2.4 mg once weekly during a 20-week run-in period were then randomized to continue

Some Contraindications/Precautions
► Contraindications ▪ Pregnancy ▪ Uncontrolled hypertension ▪ Seizure disorder or history of seizures ▪ Bulimia or anorexia nervosa ▪ Chronic opiate use or acute opiate withdrawal ▪ Within 14 days of a MAOI ► Precautions ▪ Can lower seizure threshold ▪ Suicidal thoughts/behavior ▪ Serious neuropsychiatric reactions
► Contraindications ▪ Pregnancy (when used for weight loss) ▪ Personal or family history of medullary thyroid cancer or multiple endocrine neoplasia syndrome type 2 ► Precautions ▪ Thyroid C-cell tumors ▪ Cholelithiasis ▪ Hypoglycemia ▪ Acute kidney injury ▪ Acute hypersensitivity reactions ▪ Diabetic retinopathy complications ▪ Tachycardia ▪ Suicidal ideation

semaglutide treatment or switch to placebo for 48 weeks; mean weight loss was significantly greater with semaglutide than with placebo.[20-23]

Liraglutide vs Semaglutide – A randomized, open-label, 68-week trial (STEP 8) in 338 adults without diabetes and a BMI ≥30 kg/m^2 or ≥27 and at least one weight-related comorbidity compared subcutaneous injections of semaglutide 2.4 mg once weekly and liraglutide 3 mg once daily, both in addition to diet and exercise. Mean weight loss from baseline was significantly greater with semaglutide than with liraglutide, and

Table 5. Liraglutide vs Semaglutide[1]		
Maintenance Regimen	**Mean Weight Change (%)[2]**	**% of Patients with ≥10% Weight Loss**
Liraglutide 3 mg SC once/day	-6.4%	25.6%
Semaglutide 2.4 mg SC once/week	-15.8%*	70.9%*

*Statistically significant difference vs liraglutide
1. DR Rubino et al. JAMA 2022; 327:138.
2. Mean change in body weight from baseline to week 68 in adults with a BMI ≥30 or ≥27 and at least one weight-related comorbidity.

semaglutide was associated with a greater likelihood of achieving ≥10% weight loss compared to liraglutide (see Table 5). Treatment discontinuation occurred less often with semaglutide than with liraglutide (13.5% vs 28%).[24]

In a post-hoc analysis of GLP-1 randomized controlled trials, weight loss was 11.4% with semaglutide and 4.7% with liraglutide. Semaglutide was also associated with a lower rate of discontinuation due to adverse effects.[5]

Both liraglutide and semaglutide have been shown to improve cardiovascular outcomes in patients with type 2 diabetes; cardiovascular outcome data are not yet available for either drug in patients without type 2 diabetes.

Adverse Effects – GI adverse effects, including nausea, vomiting, diarrhea, constipation, and abdominal pain, are common with GLP-1 receptor agonists. Acute pancreatitis, cholelithiasis, acute renal failure, increased heart rate, and serious hypersensitivity reactions, including angioedema and anaphylaxis, have also occurred. A meta-analysis found an association between use of GLP-1 receptor agonists, especially in high doses and for longer durations, and gall bladder and biliary diseases.[25] Contraindications to their use are listed in Table 4.

Drug Interactions – By slowing gastric emptying, GLP-1 receptor agonists can delay the absorption of oral drugs in the small intestine.

TIRZEPATIDE — In an open-label trial, 1879 patients with type 2 diabetes were randomized to receive 5, 10, or 15 mg of tirzepatide, an investigational dual glucose-dependent insulinotropic polypeptide (GIP) and GLP-1 receptor agonist, or semaglutide 1 mg injected subcutaneously once weekly (the dosage of semaglutide approved for weight loss is 2.4 mg) for 40 weeks. Reductions in body weight were significantly greater with tirzepatide than with semaglutide (-7.6 kg, -9.3 kg, and -11.2 kg, respectively, vs -5.7 kg).[26]

In an unpublished double-blind trial (SURMOUNT-1), 2539 obese or overweight adults without type 2 diabetes who had at least one weight-related comorbidity were randomized to receive tirzepatide 5, 10, or 15 mg or placebo injected subcutaneously once weekly for 72 weeks. According to the manufacturer, reductions in body weight were greater with tirzepatide than with placebo (-16 kg [16.0%], -22 kg [21.4%], -24 kg [22.5%] vs 2 kg). About 85% of patients who received the 5-mg dose and about 90% of those who received the 10- or 15-mg dose achieved ≥5% weight loss compared to 35% of those who received placebo.

PREGNANCY — All weight-loss drugs are contraindicated for use during pregnancy or breastfeeding.

DEVICES

GASTRIC ASPIRATION DEVICE — The *AspireAssist* device, which was the most effective device for weight loss, was discontinued by the manufacturer in April 2022 for financial reasons.[27]

INTRAGASTRIC BALLOON DEVICES — Two intragastric balloon devices (*Obalon Balloon System* and *Orbera Intragastric Balloon System*) are FDA-approved for up to 6 months' use in adults with a BMI ≥30 kg/m^2 who have been unable to lose or maintain weight with diet and exercise. Both devices are left in place for 6 months and then deflated and removed endoscopically. In general, they decrease caloric intake by increasing satiety/fullness. Intragastric balloon devices produce weight loss of 4-13% compared to controls and appear to be superior to diet

Table 6. Some Devices for Weight Management[1]

Device	Indication
Orbera	BMI ≥30 kg/m² if lifestyle modification is unsuccessful
Obalon	BMI ≥30 kg/m² if lifestyle modification is unsuccessful
Plenity	BMI of 25-40 kg/m² as an adjunct to diet and exercise

1. The *AspireAssist* device was discontinued by the manufacturer in April 2022.

and lifestyle modification at 6 months.[28] Liquid-filled balloons *(Orbera)* appear to produce more weight loss than gas-filled balloons *(Obalon)*, but they have a higher incidence of adverse effects.[29] Balloon devices have not been compared directly to one another or to pharmacologic or surgical methods of weight loss. Weight regain has occurred with all devices.

Orbera – The *Orbera* device is an endoscopically inserted single gastric balloon filled with up to 700 mL of saline.[30] A meta-analysis of studies assessing the *Orbera* device found a mean weight loss of 13.2% at 6 months and declining efficacy (weight regain) after that in the small number of studies reporting out to 12 and 36 months.[31] A short-term randomized controlled trial favored *Orbera* over a sham procedure with sibutramine (additional 2 kg weight loss with *Orbera*), but a long-term follow-up found no significant differences in weight loss with *Orbera* compared to controls at 2 years and 10 years.[32]

Obalon – The *Obalon Balloon System* is a gas-inflated system that uses up to three deflated balloons swallowed as capsules attached to an inflation catheter at ≥14-day intervals.[33] The catheter is used to inflate the balloons,

Mechanism of Action	Advantages and Disadvantages
Liquid-filled balloon that is endoscopically placed and removed	More weight loss compared to gas-filled balloon (13% vs 7% in 6 months), but higher rates of adverse events.
Balloon that is swallowed without requiring endoscopy, filled with gas through a catheter, and removed endoscopically	Pooled analysis found minimal benefit compared to lifestyle modification.
Superabsorbent oral hydrogel capsules that expand in the stomach to promote satiety	Minimal weight loss compared to lifestyle modification with data available from only one randomized clinical trial. Favorable safety profile.

without endoscopy or sedation, with a nitrogen sulfur-hexafluoride gas mixture and is then withdrawn. In a randomized trial in 387 patients, those who received the gas-filled intragastric balloon lost significantly more weight at 6 months than sham-treated patients (-7.1% vs -3.6%).[34]

Adverse Effects – Intragastric balloon devices have been associated with nausea, emesis, abdominal pain, reflux symptoms, and abdominal distension/bloating. If they deflate and migrate, they can cause GI obstruction. Gastric ulceration and esophageal perforation can occur. A post-approval study of the *Orbera* device found reports of hyperinflation, acute pancreatitis, and death since the device was approved in 2015. The FDA has received no reports of hyperinflation, acute pancreatitis, or death with the gas-filled *Obalon* system.[35]

Contraindications – Intragastric balloon devices are contraindicated for use in patients with a wide variety of GI conditions, including prior abdominal or weight reduction surgery, inflammatory bowel disease, obstructive disorders, GI ulcers, intestinal varices, stricture, or stenosis, severe reflux, prior GI bleeding, severe liver disease, and coagulopathy.

NONSYSTEMICALLY ABSORBED HYDROGEL — *Plenity*, a nonsystemic oral superabsorbent hydrogel formulation of cellulose and citric acid, was cleared by the FDA in 2019 for use as an adjunct to diet and exercise in overweight and obese adults (BMI of 25-40 kg/m^2). *Plenity* is the first ingested, transient, space-occupying hydrogel to be marketed in the US and the only weight management treatment available by prescription for patients with a BMI of 25-40, regardless of comorbidities (orlistat is available over the counter for the same indication).[36] Self-administered with water before lunch and dinner, *Plenity* capsules form a three-dimensional matrix that mixes with ingested food to create a sensation of fullness. The gel matrix is digested and broken down in the colon, and the particles are eliminated in feces.

In one clinical trial in 436 patients with a BMI ≥27 who were also counseled on diet and exercise, mean weight loss at 24 weeks was greater with *Plenity* than with placebo (-6.4% vs -4.4%), and more patients taking *Plenity* achieved ≥5% weight loss (59% vs 42%).[37]

Adverse Effects – GI adverse effects such as diarrhea, abdominal distension, and infrequent bowel movements are common; *Plenity* should be used with caution in patients with active GI conditions such as gastroesophageal reflux disease (GERD) or ulcers and should be avoided in patients who have GI motility issues or suspected strictures (e.g., Crohn's disease).

PREGNANCY — All weight-loss devices are contraindicated for use during pregnancy.

1. KH Lewis et al. Safety and effectiveness of longer-term phentermine use: clinical outcomes from an electronic health record cohort. Obesity (Silver Spring) 2019; 27:591.
2. DB Allison et al. Controlled-release phentermine/topiramate in severely obese adults: a randomized controlled trial (EQUIP). Obesity (Silver Spring) 2012; 20:330.
3. KM Gadde et al. Effects of low-dose, controlled-release, phentermine plus topiramate combination on weight and associated comorbidities in overweight and obese adults (CONQUER): a randomised, placebo-controlled, phase 3 trial. Lancet 2011; 377:1341.
4. WT Garvey et al. Two-year sustained weight loss and metabolic benefits with controlled-release phentermine/topiramate in obese and overweight adults (SEQUEL): a randomized, placebo-controlled, phase 3 extension study. Am J Clin Nutr 2012; 95:297.

5. Q Shi et al. Pharmacotherapy for adults with overweight and obesity: a systematic review and network meta-analysis of randomized controlled trials. Lancet 2022; 399:259.

6. AS Kelly et al. Phentermine/topiramate for the treatment of adolescent obesity. NEJM Evid 2022 April 30 (epub).

7. KM Gadde et al. Obesity: pathophysiology and management. J Am Coll Cardiol 2018; 71:69.

8. P Hollander et al. Effects of naltrexone sustained-release/bupropion sustained-release combination therapy on body weight and glycemic parameters in overweight and obese patients with type 2 diabetes. Diabetes Care 2013; 36:4022.

9. Contrave – a combination of bupropion and naltrexone for weight loss. Med Lett Drugs Ther 2014; 56:112.

10. A Siebenhofer et al. Long-term effects of weight-reducing drugs in people with hypertension. Cochrane Database Syst Rev 2021; 1:CD007654.

11. Inhibitors and inducers of CYP enzymes, P-glycoprotein, and other transporters. Med Lett Drugs Ther 2021 October 20 (epub). Available at: medicalletter.org/downloads/CYP_PGP_Tables.pdf.

12. Liraglutide (Victoza) for type 2 diabetes. Med Lett Drugs Ther 2010; 52:25.

13. Liraglutide (Saxenda) for weight loss. Med Lett Drugs Ther 2015; 57:89.

14. MJ Davies et al. Efficacy of liraglutide for weight loss among patients with type 2 diabetes: the SCALE diabetes randomized clinical trial. JAMA 2015; 314:687.

15. X Pi-Sunyer et al. A randomized, controlled trial of 3.0 mg of liraglutide in weight management. N Engl J Med 2015; 373:11.

16. TA Wadden et al. Weight maintenance and additional weight loss with liraglutide after low-calorie-diet-induced weight loss: the SCALE maintenance randomized study. Int J Obes (Lond) 2013; 37:1443.

17. CW le Roux et al. 3 years of liraglutide versus placebo for type 2 diabetes risk reduction and weight management in individuals with prediabetes: a randomised, double-blind trial. Lancet 2017; 389:1399.

18. JR Lundgren et al. Healthy weight loss maintenance with exercise, liraglutide, or both combined. N Engl J Med 2021; 384:1719.

19. Semaglutide (Wegovy) for weight loss. Med Lett Drugs Ther 2021; 63:106.

20. JPH Wilding et al. Once-weekly semaglutide in adults with overweight or obesity. N Engl J Med 2021; 384:989.

21. TA Wadden et al. Effect of subcutaneous semaglutide vs placebo as an adjunct to intensive behavioral therapy on body weight in adults with overweight or obesity: the STEP 3 randomized clinical trial. JAMA 2021; 325:1403.

22. D Rubino et al. Effect of continued weekly subcutaneous semaglutide vs placebo on weight loss maintenance in adults with overweight or obesity: the STEP 4 randomized clinical trial. JAMA 2021; 325:1414.

23. M Davies et al. Semaglutide 2.4 mg once a week in adults with overweight or obesity, and type 2 diabetes (STEP 2): a randomised, double-blind, double-dummy, placebo-controlled, phase 3 trial. Lancet 2021; 397:971.

24. DM Rubino et al. Effect of weekly subcutaneous semaglutide vs daily liraglutide on body weight in adults with overweight or obesity without diabetes: the STEP 8 randomized clinical trial. JAMA 2022; 327:138.

25. L He et al. Association of glucagon-like peptide-1 receptor agonist use with risk of gallbladder and biliary diseases: a systematic review and meta-analysis of randomized clinical trials. JAMA Intern Med 2022 Mar 28 (epub).

26. JP Frias et al. Tirzepatide versus semaglutide once weekly in patients with type 2 diabetes. N Engl J Med 2021; 385:503.

27. AspireAssist – a new device for weight loss. Med Lett Drugs Ther 2016; 58:109.

28. T Muniraj et al. AGA clinical practice guidelines on intragastric balloons in the management of obesity. Gastroenterology 2021; 160:1799.

29. AA Saber et al. Efficacy of first-time intragastric balloon in weight loss: a systematic review and meta-analysis of randomized controlled trials. Obes Surg 2017; 27:277.

30. ReShape and Orbera – two gastric balloon devices for weight loss. Med Lett Drugs Ther 2015; 57:122.

31. BK Abu Dayyeh et al. ASGE Bariatric Endoscopy Task Force systematic review and meta-analysis assessing the ASGE PIVI thresholds for adopting endoscopic bariatric therapies. Gastrointest Endosc 2015; 82:425.

32. DL Chan et al. Outcomes with intra-gastric balloon therapy in BMI <35 non-morbid obesity: 10-year follow-up study of an RCT. Obes Surg 2021; 31:781.

33. Obalon Balloon System – another gastric balloon for weight loss. Med Lett Drugs Ther 2017; 59:102.

34. S Sullivan et al. Randomized sham-controlled trial of the 6-month swallowable gas-filled intragastric balloon system for weight loss. Surg Obes Relat Dis 2018; 14:1876.

35. FDA. Update: potential risks with liquid-filled intragastric balloons – letter to health care providers. April 27, 2020. https://bit.ly/3uVOZFv. Accessed May 12, 2022.

36. Plenity for weight management. Med Lett Drugs Ther 2021; 63:77.

37. FL Greenway et al. A randomized, double-blind, placebo-controlled study of Gelesis100: a novel nonsystemic oral hydrogel for weight loss. Obesity (Silver Spring) 2019; 27:205.

Index

Index

Index

Index

Index

Index

Ritonavir
  drug interactions with, 82
Rivaroxaban, 195, 196, 199, **200**, 202, 205, 206, **208**
Rivastigmine, 47, 48, 50, **54**
Rosiglitazone, 72
Rosuvastatin, 110, 114
Rosuvastatin/ezetimibe. *See* Ezetimibe/rosuvastatin
Roszet. See Ezetimibe/rosuvastatin
Roxybond. See Oxycodone
Rybelsus. See Semaglutide for type 2 diabetes

S

Sabal serrulatum, 43
Salicylates. *See also* individual drug names
  for pain, **131**
Salsalate, 132, 134
Sarcoptes scabiei, 189
Savaysa. See Edoxaban
Savella. See Milnacipran
Saw palmetto
  for BPH, 43
Saxagliptin, 71, 72, 76, 83
Saxagliptin/dapagliflozin. *See* Dapagliflozin/saxagliptin
Saxagliptin/metformin, 78
Saxenda. See Liraglutide for weight management
Scabies, drugs for, 180, 189
Seglentis. See Tramadol/celecoxib
Segluromet. See Ertugliflozin/metformin
Selective serotonin reuptake inhibitors. *See also* individual drug names
  for dementia, 60
  drug interactions with, 167
Semaglutide
  for type 2 diabetes, 67–71, 76, 82
  for weight management, 216, 218, **223,** 226
Serenoa repens, 43
Serologic antibody test
  for *Helicobacter pylori,* 97
Seroquel. See Quetiapine

Serotonin and norepinephrine reuptake inhibitors. *See also* individual drug names
  for pain, 130, 141, 142, **144**
Sertraline
  for dementia, 60
Sexually transmitted infections, drugs for, **173**
Shingles. *See* Zoster vaccine
Shingrix. See Zoster vaccine
Silodosin, 35, 36
Simvastatin, 108, 109, 114
Simvastatin/ezetimibe. *See* Ezetimibe/simvastatin
Sinecathechins
  for STIs, 180, 189
Sitagliptin, 66, 67, 71, 72, 76, 83
Sitagliptin/metformin, 78
Slo-Niacin. See Niacin
SNRIs. *See* Serotonin and norepinephrine reuptake inhibitors
Sodium bicarbonate/omeprazole. *See* Omeprazole/sodium bicarbonate
Solifenacin, 38, 42
Soliqua. See Insulin glargine/lixisenatide
Soliris. See Eculizumab
Sprix. See Ketorolac
SSRIs. *See* Selective serotonin reuptake inhibitors
Staphylococcus aureus, 1
Statins, **107,** 123
Steglatro. See Ertugliflozin
Steglujan. See Ertugliflozin/sitagliptin
STEP 1-4, 222
STEP 8, 227
STIs. *See* Sexually transmitted infections
Stool antigen test, 96, 97
Streptococcus pneumoniae, 1–3
Stromectol. See Ivermectin
Subsys. See Fentanyl
Sucralfate
  for PUD, 94, 101, 102
SURMOUNT-1, 229
Symproic, 152

Index